T0319015

Nutrition and health of the gastrointestinal tract

Nutrition and health

of the

gastrointestinal tract

Editors:

M.C. Blok

H.A. Vahl

L. de Lange

A.E. van de Braak

G. Hemke

M. Hessing

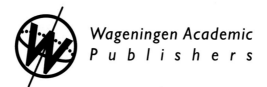

Wageningen Academic
Publishers

CIP-data Koninklijke Bibliotheek
Den Haag

ISBN 9076998116   paperback

Subject headings:
animals
gastrointestinal tract
health
nutrition
First published, 2002

Illustration cover:
Scanning Electron Microscopical
reproduction of intestinal villi.
By courtesy of Department of
Pathology, Faculty Veterinary Medicine,
Utrecht University

Wageningen Academic Publishers
The Netherlands, 2002

Printed in The Netherlands

Contents

Preface

Today, one of the main interests within animal nutrition is the relation between nutrition and gut health, especially that of the small intestine.

In the Netherlands, the Product Board Animal Feed, a public organisation of interest for all concerns within the feed chain, is one of the main national financiers of research projects in this field. As a financier interested in funding research with resultswhich will be applicable in practice, the Board was confronted with the question of which type of projects were the most promising to subsidise.

The Board has been subsidising research projects in the field of animal nutrition for many years. In the period 1980 - 1995, most attention was paid to research which aimed to improve the efficiency of animal production and to lower the costs of animal nutrition. After financing many projects which aimed to reduce the excretion of nitrogen and phosphorus to the environment (an important issue in the Netherlands since the mid-eighties), the Board decided some years ago that research dealing with the theme 'animal nutrition and health of the gastrointestinal tract', especially in young animals, need to be stimulated.

Research concerning the role of animal nutrition on gut health has already been stimulated by the fact that Dutch farmers and the feed industry have to take into account a (total) ban in the European Union, of anti-microbial growth promoters as additives in animal nutrition within a couple of years. This forthcoming ban particularly stimulated research focussed on 'the management of the micro-flora' by a change in the composition of the animal feed.

About a year ago, the Board decided that for future financing of nutritional research dealing with the relation nutrition to gut health, a more comprehensive insight in the effects of nutrition on gastrointestinal health was urgently required. Therefore it was decided to organise a workshop, that would concentrate on the following questions:
- What is a physiologically healthy gut?
- What is an optimal micro-flora?
- What qualifies as good integrity and functionality of the intestinal wall?
- What is the ideal status of the immune system in the gut wall?
- Which available methods and techniques to study these aspects, are reliable, reproducible and have predictable power?
- What is known already and what can be expected concerning the role of (adapted) animal nutrition?

This workshop was held in the summer of 2001. The organisers (and editors of this book) felt that the various scientific contributions to this workshop were of interest to a much broader public, and so it was decided to publish the lectures.

In the introductory chapter, the authors dealwith the question of when it can be concluded that an animal has a healthy gut. Subsequently there are three disciplinary chapters concentrating on the importance of the micro-flora, the integrity and functionality of the gut wall, and the immune system. Attention is paid also to a number of techniques and methods to study these functions and to several important aspects of nutrition.

In the second part of the workshop three cases, dealing with different health problems in different species were highlighted. Special attention was paid to: the role of nutrition in post weaning edema disease in piglets, the (potential) importance of feed components in *Eimeria* infections in chickens, and the consequences of replacement of milk protein by vegetable protein in milk replacer diets for veal calves.

Together these chapters give an interesting and well documented overview of the present state of the art with respect to the most important aspects of gut health and the importance of nutrition on these functions. Although no clear-cut conclusions could be made, the Board concluded that the workshop has yielded a number of important elements for future decisions to finance research in this area.

1. Optimising nutrient digestion, absorption and gut barrier function in monogastrics: Reality or illusion?

J.D. van der Klis and A.J.M. Jansman
ID TNO Animal Nutrition, PO Box 65, NL 8200 AB, Lelystad

1.1. Introduction

Nutritionists and feed manufacturers are becoming increasingly aware of the fact that the major gut functions, digestion, absorption and intestinal barrier (as the first line of defence against invasive pathogens) in monogastrics should be optimised to achieve a high production performance, at minimal nutrient use for immune or anti-inflammatory responses. Nutrient expenditure for immune responses are high, as demonstrated by Klasing and Calvert (1998) for poultry and by Huisman (1999) for pigs (after Stahly, 1996).

It is evident that the use of poorly degradable feed components will reduce animal performance due to a low nutrient absorption and thus a limited nutrient availability for production purposes. On the other hand, feed components being resistant to enzymatic degradation serve as a substrate for bacterial activity in the intestinal lumen. The interaction between host nutrition and the intestinal microbiota has been clearly illustrated using germ-free animals. For example, Langhout (1998) showed that the antinutritional effects of highly methylated citrus pectin were small or even absent in germ-free broiler chickens, while production performance, and especially fat digestibility, were clearly reduced in conventionally raised broiler chickens. Control of the activity of the small intestinal microbiota is important to avoid undesired competition for nutrients between bacteria and the host animal and to restrict bacterial overgrowth. Of course, positive effects of microbial metabolites should not be neglected. Short chain fatty acids are a source of energy to the host animal, can inhibit growth of pathogens, can improve epithelial cell proliferation and stimulate immune competence.

Gut health is challenged during animal growth at different occasions, e.g. at weaning of piglets, during climate stress, or after infections with bacterial pathogens or viruses.

In this paper several examples of research models to study different aspects of gut health are briefly outlined. Some parameters or characteristics of the health status of the gut are considered. It should be accentuated, however, that these characteristics or measurements are derived from a variety of experiments with different aims e.g. being addressed to study microbial fermentation, intestinal integrity, barrier function, and/or immune responsiveness (ter Huurne et al., 2000). Studies in which different gut health parameters are related to production performance are needed to be able to predict the importance of different health aspects and correlate those with a loss in production performance during a state of compromised gut health. So far such studies are scarce.

1.2. Response criteria and normal values

In the literature many response criteria have been used to describe gastrointestinal health. These parameters have been summarised in Table 1 (as mean values plus standard error). In general only a limited number of parameters is considered per study. Therefore, often data do not enable calculation of mutual correlations between parameters or with production performance. If data from Table 1 are affected by for instance age, strain, or feed intake, effects have been described later in this chapter.

1.3. Intestinal weight and length

Postnatal development of the gastrointestinal tract in pigs and poultry follows an allometric growth curve (Lilja, 1983; Kelly, 1994). During the first 12 days of life, the weights of the proximal parts of the small intestine (duodenum and jejunum) increase in mass more rapidly than distal segments (ileum) in broiler chickens. Uni et al. (1999) observed a 2- to 4-fold increase in intestinal length up to 12 days of age, while the weight of these segments increased 7- to 10-fold. They found a maximum relative intestinal weight of the small intestine at 5 to 7 days of age. From that age, the rate of gain of total body weight exceeded that of the gastrointestinal tract, resulting in a reduction in the relative weight of the latter.

In broilers, length and weight of the small intestine increase when diets are fed with lower digestibilities (Smits, 1996). He observed an increase in length and weight of the small intestine from 3.9 to 5.3 g and 13.4 to 16.8 cm (all expressed per 100 g BW), when a low and highly methylated CMC were included in corn/soy diets from 3 to 5 weeks of age. It is well-documented that feeding poorly enzymatically digestible, but highly fermentable diets to broilers and pigs results in an increased intestinal length and thicker intestinal wall, and consequently in an increase in relative volume and intestinal weight. Brenes et al. (1993) found an increased pancreatic weight when poorly digestible diets were fed to broilers. A similar relationship between dietary content of fermentable carbohydrates and size/weight of the gastrointestinal tract or pancreas weight was documented for pigs (Drochner, 1993). Data from Simon (2001) indicated a clear increase in the relative weight of the intestinal tract of broilers with increasing digesta viscosities (Figure 1). Van der Klis et al. (1999) showed a high negative correlation (r=-0.98) between growth rate from 0 to 3 weeks of age and the intestinal weight in broiler chickens fed diets with different NSP sources. This negative correlation reflects data in Figure 1.

Table 1. Normal[1] values of gastrointestinal parameters or health-related parameters measured in poultry and pigs.

	Poultry		Pigs	
	mean	s.e.	mean	s.e.
Digestion				
Enzyme activity lumen				
Trypsin (duodenum), U/g dm chyme	-		200-600	182
Trypsin (jejunum), U/g dm chyme	-		250-425	72
Chymotrypsin (duodenum), U/g dm chyme	-		25-85	24
Chymotrypsin (jejunum), U/g dm chyme	-		33-50	7
Enzyme activity brush border				
Sucrase, U/g	156	35	760	102
Maltase, U/g	944	224	210	34
Alkaline phosphatase, U/g	116	24	-	
Glutamyletransferase, U/g	1790	320	-	
Absorption				
Morphometry[1]				
Villous height (jejunum), μm	612	61	400-550	35
Crypt depth (jejunum), μm	188	25	170-210	14
Villous width (jejunum), μm	111	16	-	
Enterocytes per villus	848	189	-	
Enterocytes per μm villus	1.34	0.13	-	
Barrier function				
Mucus production (U/g chyme)	15		-	
Permeability coefficient (mannitol, 10^{-6}cm/sec)	5	1.5	6.5-8.0	0.9
Physico-chemical conditions				
pH, duodenum	5.5-6.2		5.5-6.7	
pH, jejunum	5.8-6.9		6.0-8.00	
pH, ileum	6.3-8.0		6.6-8.0	
Viscosity, jejunum, mPa.s	1.2-10.0		-	
Viscosity, ileum, mPa.s	1.2-23.7		-	
Retention time, jejunum, min	71-84		100	
Retention time, ileum, min	90-97		-	
Others				
Microbial activity				
ATP concentration (jejunum), mmol/l	1.9	0.5	2	
ATP concentration (ileum) mmol/l	4.3	1.3	4-9	
VFA concentration (small intestine), mmol/kg	7.8-25.5		1.4-2.5	0.3
Bile salt concentration (small intestine), μmol/g	11.7-14.4		-	
Bacterial translocation				
NO x (μmol/l blood serum)[z]	10.1	0.6	-	

[1]Normal values refer to values in a healthy intestinal tract

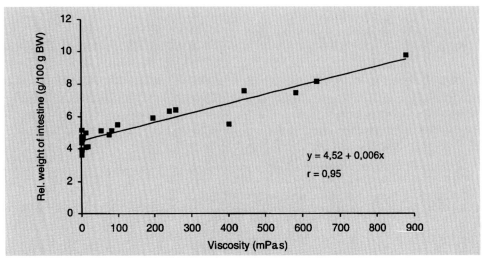

Figure 1. Relationship between the viscosity of digesta in the jejunum and the relative weight of the intestinal tissue of broilers (Simon, 2001).

Extreme intraluminal viscosities as indicated in Figure 1 are not realistic under practical feeding conditions, but an increase in relative intestinal weight of 30% can be found in both broilers and pigs (Simon, 2001 after Jørgensen, 1996).

1.4. Morphological and secretory development of the intestinal tract

In turkey poults, pancreatic enzyme activities (like trypsin, protease and amylase) in digesta in the intestines increase during the first three weeks of life, whereas lipase activity remains constant (Krogdahl and Sell, 1989). A similar pattern was observed in broiler chickens (Noy and Sklan, 1995). Nitsan et al. (1991) indicated that lipase could be limiting for fat digestion during the first two weeks of age in broiler chickens. Moreover, the presence or lack of bile acids also affects fat digestibility. In broilers and in pigs, the primary bile acids are chenodeoxycholyltauric and cholyltauric acid (Elkin et al., 1990). Secreted bile acids are readily absorbed from the small intestine and recirculate for 90% (Hurwitz et al., 1973). In young broilers bile acid production is limited (Green and Kellogg, 1987), which limits fat digestion. This is particularly clear for saturated fatty acids.

Age patterns in enzyme activity in young poults resemble those in piglets. Development of the pancreas and its proteolytic enzymes in pigs in time is presented in Table 2. It is clear that pancreatic enzyme activities increase especially during the first 20 days of age.

During the postnatal development in pigs a gradual shift in intestinal digestive enzymes (decline in lactase and increase in maltase and sucrase), gastric secretions,

Table 2. Age-related changes in the pancreas and activities of trypsin, carboxypeptidase A (CPA) and carboxypeptidase B (CPB) in piglets from birth to 30 days of age (after Tarvid et al., 1994).

Age (days)	Neonatal	2	10	20	30
BW (kg)	1.04	1.64	3.62	7.13	10.41
Pancreas (g)	1.04	2.46	5.31	8.54	11.21
Protein in pancreas (mg)	128	271	800	1322	1799
Trypsin (U/gland)	22.2	48.3	74.7	117.9	284.7
Chymotrypsin (U/gland)	5.8	12.9	22.6	37.8	46.0
CPA (U/gland)	2.4	6.1	18.6	24.4	21.6
CPB (U/gland)	2.8	8.0	22.2	43.6	43.7

and volumes of pancreatic-biliary secretions is observed (Pierzynowski et al., 1995). They found that the pancreatic secretion in suckling piglets was low (less than 1 ml/kg BW/h) compared to the postweaning period (1.5 to 2.5 ml/kg BW/h). These differences will partly be due to source and level of dietary proteins and other nutrients (e.g. organic acids) which may modify the volume of pancreatic juice and (or) activities of pancreatic/intestinal enzymes in weaned piglets.

1.4.1. Brush border enzyme activities

Uni et al. (1999) described the development of the intestinal morphology and function with age in broilers. They observed a close correlation between the duodenal mucosal sucrase and glucosyltransferase (brush border enzyme involved in amino acid transport) enzyme activities per g wet tissue and the numbers of enterocytes per villus ($r^2>0.90$). The correlations between the morphological parameters in the ileum and the activity of maltase and alkaline phosphatase in all intestinal segments were much lower. Others established that mature and active enterocytes express disaccharidase and alkaline phosphatase activities (Weiser, 1973). Uni et al. (1999) also showed a close correlation between the mucosal enzyme activities (sucrase, maltase and glutamyletransferase) and the body weight of broilers from 1 to 12 days of age, while alkaline phosphatase showed lower correlation values.

In chicks, villous height and crypt depth increased rapidly after hatch and reached a plateau in 6 d in de duodenum and 10 d in the jejunum and ileum. Villous height and crypt depth measurements in piglets reared under various conditions were reported by Nabuurs (1991). In Table 3 a comparison among three herds is presented: 1) herds with a history of postweaning diarrhoea (PWD) without mortality; 2) SPF herd and 3) PWD herd with mortality. It was shown that in herds with mortality villus height was clearly reduced compared to herds without mortality and SPF herds, while crypt depth was increased in both PWD herds compared to the SPF herd.

Table 3. A comparative study of villous height and crypt depth measurements in piglets from three herds, differing in health status (after Nabuurs, 1991).

Days after weaning	PWD herds without mortality	SPF herd	PWD herd with mortality
Villous height (µm)			
0	375[b]	425[a]	175[c]
4	350[a]	340[a]	160[b]
7	350[a]	375[a]	160[b]
11	360[b]	450[a]	155[c]
14	400[b]	500[a]	155[c]
Crypt depth (µm)			
0	175[a]	25[b]	155[a]
4	180[a]	60[b]	160[a]
7	215[a]	150[b]	245[a]
11	225[a]	150[b]	200[a]
14	265[a]	150[b]	225[a]

1.5. Development of the intestinal microbiota

At hatching of broilers or birth of piglets the gastrointestinal tract is sterile. Immediately bacteria, originating from the mother, the environment, or the diet will colonise in the GI tract. In case of mother contacts, a diverse microbial population will enter the GI tract. As a result after the first colonisation, new bacterial species will have more difficulties to colonise (colonisation resistance). Because of the strict separation of generations in broiler chickens, any bacteria from the environment might colonise (e.g. attach to intestinal binding sites or multiply faster than being removed via chyme passage) in the intestinal tract. To overcome the vulnerability for colonisation of potential pathogens, competitive exclusion products (often being a microbiota of healthy adult animals) can be used. Using such products will shorten the period needed to establish a stable microbiota. Once solid food is digested, obligate anaerobes increase in number and diversity, especially in the hindgut. The composition of the microbiota varies in different parts of the gastrointestinal tract, as shown for pigs in Figure 2 (Jensen, 1999).

In the proximal parts of the GI tract (crop and stomach), lactobacilli and streptococci are abundantly present, which is believed to be associated with the specific epithelial surface in these proximal gastrointestinal segments (Tannock, 1990 as cited by Jensen, 1999). A substantial microbial fermentation takes place in the crop of poultry and in the stomach of pigs (Jensen, 1999). As the pH in the gizzard of poultry is much lower than in the stomach of pigs, the duodenal microbiota is depopulated in poultry to a larger extent than in pigs. Furthermore, secreted enzymes and bile acids have a further bacteriostatic effect. In more distal parts the enzyme concentrations or activities are

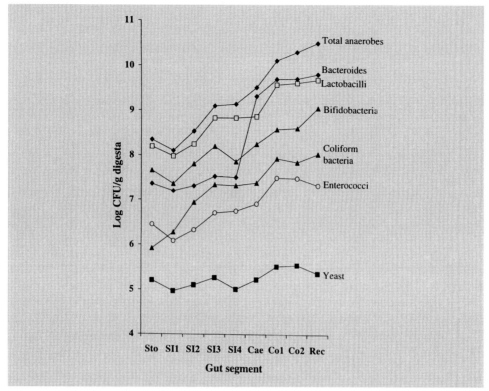

Figure 2. The density of selected populations of the microbiota in various regions of the gastrointestinal tract of pigs (originally published by Jensen, 1999).

reduced and bile acids are deconjugated or reabsorbed, which makes the environment more preferable for microbial growth.

Especially in the lower intestinal part, chyme retention time is increased (Van der Klis, 1993). This means that more time is available for bacteria to multiply, resulting in an extensive and diverse anaerobic microbial population (Jensen, 1991). Based on conventional plating techniques to culture microbial species from fresh intestinal contents, only a small fraction of all species will be identified. New techniques are available based on PCR amplification, which enables identification without culturing. Identification of the composition of the microflora has only limited value to substantiate the microbial activity.

A diverse and stabile microbiota will prevent new bacterial strains from colonisation. If digestion and absorption become compromised a larger portion of protein and starch reaches the lower intestinal parts which causes a change in microbial inhabitants and activity in broiler chickens (Wagner and Thomas, 1987). They observed that rye-based diets result in a larger anaerobic ileal population than on maize. Van der Klis et al. (1999) observed a positive correlation between the number of E. coli in the lumen of the small intestine and the AME conversion (i.e. MJ AME/kg BWG) in young

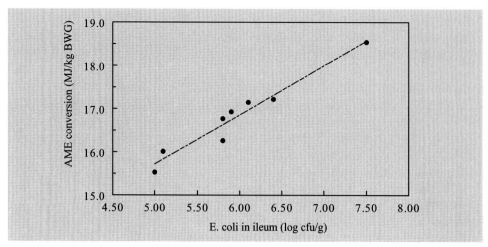

Figure 3. The relationship between the AME conversion (MJ AME intake/kg BWG) and the number of E. coli in ileal digesta (log cfu/g) in young broilers (Van der Klis et al., 1999).

broiler chickens (Figure 3). An increased AME conversion (i.e. lower nutrient utilisation) that was caused by stimulated intraluminal viscosities clearly resulted in higher numbers of intraluminal E. coli.

Jensen (1999) used the luminal ATP content to quantify the microbial activity (Figure 4). He compared the ATP concentration in various regions of the gastrointestinal tract of pigs fed either a low fibre diet as such or supplemented with oat bran or wheat bran. As clearly shown in Figure 4, the ATP concentration in the proximal segments of the gastro-intestinal tract is low and hardly affected by diet composition, while in the lower small intestine, the caeca and especially in the colon large differences in microbial activity were noticed. Values in broiler chickens are somewhat lower than in pigs. Smits (1996) observed ATP concentrations of 1.0, 2.2 and 11.2 mg/l in the jejunal, ileal and caecal contents respectively.

More recent data with broilers indicated similar values as reported in Figure 4 (as indicated in section "Microbiota-host interactions"). Despite a similar microbial composition and microbial activity data in pigs and poultry, microbial fermentation in pigs is more important than in poultry, potentially because of the longer feed passage time in pigs (especially in the lower intestinal tract) than in poultry.

Differences in activity of the microbial population have also been quantified using short chain fatty acids (SCFA) concentrations in the intestinal lumen as a response parameter. It can be questioned however, if SCFA concentrations are a good response parameter, as Carré et al. (1995) indicated that SCFA are absorbed very effectively from the gastrointestinal lumen of broilers. This was in accordance to measurements with 50-60 kg pigs fed a control diet without and with 15% sugar beet pulp (SBP) and 10% wheat bran (WB) (Jansman et al., 1998a, b). They determined the lactic acid and

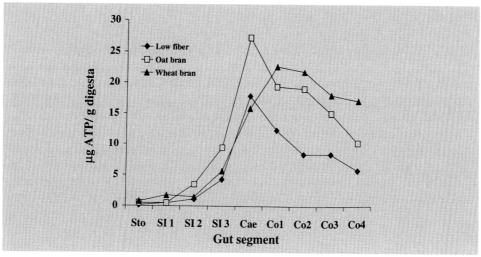

Figure 4. The microbial activity, as measured by the ATP concentration in various segments of the gastrointestinal tract of pigs. A low fibre diet was fed as such or supplemented with oat bran or wheat bran (Jensen, 1999).

propionic acid concentrations in the lower ileum and compared these concentrations with portal fluxes of these nutrients (Table 4). Dietary supplementation with SBP and WB resulted in a 50-100% increase of the lactic acid and propionic acid concentration in ileal digesta, while portal fluxes of these nutrients were increased 2- to 3-fold.

Jamroz et al. (1996) indicated that the VFA contents in the small intestine, colon and caecum of different poultry species fed corn-, barley-, or wheat-rye based diets were 7.8-25.5, 12.8-42.3 and 105-195 mmol/kg chyme, respectively. However, values obtained by Van der Klis et al. (1999) in 21-day old broilers fed corn-, wheat- or rye-based diets were substantially lower (2.3-5.8 and 49-75 mmol/kg chyme in the ileum and caeca respectively).

Table 4. The effect of fermentable fiber in pig diets on the lactic acid and propionic acid concentrations in the ileum and on portal fluxes of these nutrients (Jansman et al. 1998a, b).

	Control	Control + SBP/WB	SED
Lactic acid, mmol/kg ileal chyme	17.2	23.7	3.9
Lactic acid, portal flux, mmol/kg dm intake	263	504	60
Propionic acid, mmol/kg ileal chyme	3.1	5.8	1.0
Propionic acid, portal flux, mmol/kg dm intake	125	412	31

1.6. Microbiota - host interactions

The microbial population in the small intestinal tract competes with the host animal for nutrients. Production performance of germ-free animals on highly digestible diets exceeds performance of conventionally raised chickens (Muramatsu et al., 1994). The latter may be due to four reasons: 1) competition for nutrients; 2) lower endogenous secretions; 3) lower concentration of bacterial reaction products; and 4) better health status, which means that less nutrients are needed for immune response or acute phase reactions. However, the intestinal microbiota can also be beneficial in case of poorly digestible diets, as it will ferment indigestible feed components. In pigs, up to 30% of energy for maintenance could be retained due to microbial biodegradation, particularly in the large intestine (Drochner, 1993, Jansman et al., 2001).

1.6.1. Nutrient digestibility and availability

Nutrient availability for the animal in mostly quantified in digestibility studies with target animal species. It should be realised that such studies provide an indirect measure for the nutrient availability of the animal. First, apparent nutrient digestibilities are obtained, meaning that a significant fraction of the apparently undigested nutrients consists of endogenous constituents, being constituents that are secreted or lost in the lumen of the GI tract during the process of digestion. Only a relatively small fraction (estimated 20-35%) of the total amount of endogenous protein secreted in the GI tract is recovered at the end of the small intestine of pigs. This is true in particular for protein and amino acids. In pigs, the endogenous CP losses at the end of the terminal ileum amount 12-30 g/kg dry matter intake, depending on diet composition. Quantitative estimates for poultry are hardly found, but can be expected to fall in the same range.

In cases where the health status of the GI tract is compromised, nutrient digestibility can be reduced as a result of a reduced secretion or activity of digestive enzymes, an increased secretion of endogenous constituents (i.c. proteins) or a reduced recycling of endogenous protein. Moreover, the maintenance requirement of the GI tract can be increased under conditions of a suboptimal gastro intestinal health. Simon (2001) estimated that GI tract tissue weight in broilers could increase by 30%, when feeding diets with a high level of structural carbohydrates or highly viscous diets. It was estimated that due to the higher weight and the relatively high protein turnover rate of the GI tract, relative to protein in other tissues, an increase of 5% in total heat production is possible. This has to be considered as energy losses associated with the response of the GI system towards the diet (Table 5).

Nyachotti et al. (1997) estimated the energetic costs of synthesising endogenous gut proteins due to dietary trypsin inhibitors, as found in legume seeds. These calculations (Table 6) were based on data for the endogenous N losses in piglets as measured by Schulze (1994). The energetic costs for protein synthesis were estimated at 4.5 kJ per g of protein and the daily maintenance requirement for ME of a piglet of 13 kg BW was assumed to be 460 kJ per $kg^{0.75}$.

Table 5. Model calculation in broiler chickens for the effect of a 30% increase in the amount of protein in the gastrointestinal tissue (GIT) on energy metabolism (calculated for 1 kg BW). Calculations made by Simon (2001).

	Amount of protein (g)	Fractional synthesis rate (%/day)	Amount of protein synthesised (g/day)	GIT 130%
Total body	160	23	36.8	39.2
Skeletal muscles	88	10	8.8	8.8
GIT	11.2	70	7.8	10.2
Heat production (kJ/d)		625+30 kJ (GIT 130%)= 5% increase		

Table 6. Estimated energy costs for synthesising endogenous proteins in a 13 kg piglet fed a corn starch-based, semi-synthetic diet supplemented with graded levels of trypsin inhibitors.

Trypsin inhibitor level[1] (mg/kg)	Excreted ileal endogenous N (g/day)	Total synthesised endogenous N (g/day)[2]	Energy costs of endogenous protein synthesis (kJ/day)	% of maintenance energy requirement
0	9.7	38.6	174	5.5
1.9	16.3	65.2	293	9.3
5.7	23.0	91.9	414	13.1

Adapted by Huisman (1999) after Nyachotti et al. (1997)
[1]   Trypsin inhibitor activity (TIA) expressed in mg trypsin inhibited per g diet.
[2]   Calculated on the basis of the assumption that the secretion of endogenous N is four times higher than the endogenous N losses measured at the terminal ileum (Souffrant, 1991).

Effects of NDF from wheat bran in the diet on maintenance energy requirement were smaller than for trypsin inhibitors (max 2% increase), as calculated by Huisman (1999). These data show the potential impact of responses of the gastro-intestinal system towards constituents in the diet resulting in a significant reduction of the availability of energy for production purposes. Beside the energetic costs associated with the synthesis and recycling of endogenous protein, these processes are also resulting in N- and amino acid losses, leading to a reduced availability of amino acids for net protein retention in the body of pigs (Grala, 1998).

Hylemond (1985) has shown that the intestinal microbiota deconjugate bile acids. In humans, bile acid deconjugation is used as a measure for bacterial overgrowth (Masclee et al., 1989). Especially in young animals with limited bile acid synthesis, bacterial activity may reduce fat digestibility, as bile acids are needed for fat emulsification, colipase activation and absorption of fatty acids from the small intestine (Green and Kellogg, 1987). Moreover, the reutilization of absorbed deconjugated bile acids is less effective than of conjugated bile acids, which implies that the pool size will be reduced by microbial activity in case of a limited rate of synthesis (Juste et al. 1983). Although Langhout et al. (1998) also observed clear differences in the level of deconjugation using NSP rich diets, they concluded from their results that total bile acid production in 3-week-old broilers was not affected.

1.6.2. Effects on intestinal barrier function

During microbial fermentation different metabolites are formed which can be harmful for the host animal: 1) deconjugated and dehydroxylated bile acids, 2) potentially toxic amino acid catabolites (amines, ammonia, phenols and indoles). The intestinal epithelial barrier should keep these noxious elements within the intestinal lumen. The barrier function of the epithelial lining of the intestine can be divided into a mucosa associated (extrinsic) part, for instance the mucus and unstirred water layer, which originates from the epithelium, but exert its effect in the lumen, and a barrier formed by the mucosa as such (intrinsic) (Figure 5).

The mucus gel (extrinsic barrier) is a 450 µm thick layer covering the epithelial surface (Rozee et al., 1982). This layer is also known as an unstirred water layer and affects both passive and active transport processes (Thomson and Dietschy, 1977). Its barrier function originates from covering the cellular glycolipid and glycoprotein receptors

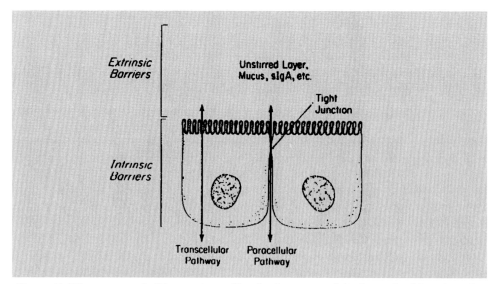

Figure 5. Diagrammatic illustration of both elements of the intestinal barrier: the extrinsic barrier, being the unstirred layer and mucus residues and the intrinsic barrier having transcellular and paracellular pathways. Tight junctions are the rate limiting step for the latter pathway (originally published by Madara et al., 1988).

on the cell surface, mimicking the cellular receptors to which bacteria attach and physically entrapment of bacteria.

Microbial metabolites stimulate the rate of proliferation and enterocyte turnover (Seidel et al., 1985; Noack et al., 1996), stimulate mucus production and reduce intestinal integrity (i.e. barrier function). A higher turnover rate of enterocytes results in less mature cells, being less capable for nutrient absorption and having more open tight junctions. In broilers, it was shown that inclusion of 2% HMC pectin in a corn-soy diet resulted in an increase of the ileal ATP concentration from 3.6 to 6.5 mg/kg contents and a fourfold increase in mucus content (from 15 to 58 relative units/g chyme) (Van der Klis, unpublished data). Dänicke (2000) has shown that the apparent digestibility of threonine (which is one of the most abundant amino acid in mucin proteins) was reduced to a larger extend than lysine with increasing intestinal viscosities. Apart from an increase in mucus production, also a shift in mucin composition was noted from sulpho to sialo type mucins. Micro-organisms can adhere to mucin receptors. Therefore, mucins play a role in both the host's mucosal line of defence and the susceptibility to infection (Helander et al., 1997). It is hypothesised that sialo type mucins are also used as a line of defence as they have less attachment sites for intestinal bacteria than sulpho type mucins. Others suggested that sialo-mucins are produced by less mature globlet cells than sulpho-mucins, which implies that the ratio between both may be a reflection of the length/maturity of the villi and crypts. Apart from effects on mucus production, also the intestinal barrier function was compromised in broilers fed corn/soy diets with 3% of HMC pectin (Van der Klis and Versantvoort, 1999). After a three-week period, the transcellular and paracellular permeability were determined at the end of the jejunum using a dipeptide (Glysar) and mannitol as markers. It was demonstrated that the paracellular permeability was increased threefold, while the transcellular permeability was not affected. As bacteria and bacterial toxins pass the intestinal mucosa primarily paracellularly, this would make the birds more vulnerable for bacterial translocation.

1.7. Research models available to study different aspects of gastrointestinal health

1.7.1. Weaning of piglets

Throughout their life, pigs face at least one initial period of feed (and water) deprivation directly after weaning. In general, weaning causes a stress reaction as manifested by an immediate reduction in feed intake, independently of dietary composition (McCracken et al., 1995). The absence of luminal stimulation and malnutrition of the enterocytes causes a reduction in villous height and increase crypt depth in the piglets (Kelly et al., 1991, Pluske et al., 1997). Verdonk et al. (1999) have shown differences in histology and integrity of the small intestinal mucosa just after weaning of piglets fed with milk at a low ($^1/_3$ of the normal, according to the daily energy requirement, intake level) versus normal intake level. They showed a clear reduction in villous height at the low level of intake, which coincided with increased paracellular permeability (Table 7). This was evident just after weaning (first two days). A similar process seems to occur in both young and older chickens. For example, in six-week-old chickens villus shortening and thickening was observed when feed intake was reduced (Michael and Hodges, 1973).

A low feed intake around weaning may also cause an increased mRNA expression of the pro-inflammatory cytokine IL-1. It was hypothesised by Verdonk (unpublished) that the integrity of the gut mucosa of piglets was compromised at the low feed intake level by an inflammatory response. This inflammatory response was manifested by villous atrophy and increased paracellular permeability, whereas at normal nutrient intakes, structure and functionality of the intestinal mucosa was maintained. The latter observation was confirmed by Spreeuwenberg et al. (2001) who demonstrated a reduced ratio of CD4/CD8 T-lymphocytes ratio in the lamina propria of the crypts at the low feed intake level after weaning. They found a reduction in this ratio from 2.2 at day 0 into 1.1 and 1.4 at day 1 and 2 respectively (SEM 0.26). At 4 days post weaning initial values were restored. Moreover, they showed a significantly positive correlation between CD8 T-cells in the lamina propria and paracellular transport rate of a marker (mannitol), which indicates a direct involvement of acute inflammation in the

Table 7. Villous length (µm), crypt depth (µm) and transcellular and paracellular transport rates ($10^{-6}.cm.s^{-1}$) in piglets fed at a high or low nutrient intake level at different time points post weaning*.

	Intestinal site	Intake level (I) High	Low	sem	Day post weaning (D) 0	1	2	4	sem	P value I	D
Villous height	proximal	465[a]	375[b]	25	502	443[a]	355[b]	409[ab]	22	*	*
	middle	370	326	22	351	382[a]	286[b]	319[b]	19	ns	**
	distal	227	212	13	255	228	207	242	11	ns	ns
Crypt depth	proximal	193	182	7	178	169[a]	172[a]	196[b]	6	ns	**
	middle	177	171	6	176	163[a]	161[a]	189[b]	5	ns	***
	distal	156	152	8	157	143	137	163	7	ns	t
Paracellular	middle	8.2[a]	12.1[b]	0.9	6.6	7.8[a]	11.4[b]	11.1[b]	0.8	**	***
Transcellular	middle	13.0	16.3	1.5	16.6	14.3	16.7	17.8	1.3	ns	ns

level of significance: ns = not significant; t = P<0.10; * P< 0.05; ** P<0.01; *** P<0.001
[abc] = Least square means in the same row without a common character in the superscript differ significantly (P<0.05).

intestinal permeability. Also Ganessunker et al. (1999) observed high negative correlations (>-0.80) between villous height and villous width to the jejunal and ileal CD4 and CD8 T-cell numbers. However, they could not ascertain whether compromised villous morphology preceded intestinal T-cell expansion or vice versa.

1.7.2. The role of the microbiota on intestinal heath parameters and bacterial translocation

The effect of the activity of the intestinal microbiota in broiler chickens can be studied using a model substance in the diet to increase the microbial activity in the intestinal tract. Langhout (1998) used 3% HMC pectin to do so. It was clearly shown by him that the presence of the intestinal microbiota mediated the antinutritive effects of HMC pectin, comparing production performance and nutrient digestibilities between conventional and germ-free broiler chickens (Table 8). Extension and optimisation of this model made clear that a higher microbial activity in the small intestine (concluded from increased ATP contents) coincided with an increased permeability of the tight junctions (Figure 6), and increased mucus contents (which is related to the higher intestinal viscosity). These data gave insight in the mode of action of the microbiota in the intestinal lumen.

1.7.3. Quantification of glucose and amino acid requirements in immune compromised animals using the insulin clamp technique

Stahly (1996) indicated that chronic immune system activation resulted in a change in efficiency and composition of growth in young pigs. Piglets (6-27 kg body weight) from the same herd were housed under conditions leading to a low or high immune

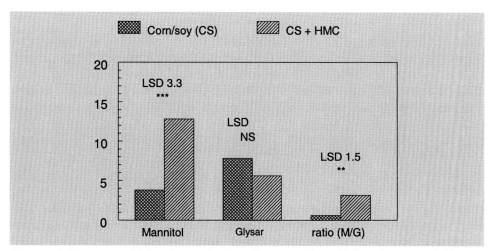

Figure 6. The paracellular (mannitol) and transcellular (glysar) permeability in broilers fed a corn/soybean meal diet with and without 3% highly methylated citrus (HMC) pectin (Van der Klis en Versantvoort, 1999).

Table 8. Production performance and nutrient digestibilities in conventional and germ-free broiler chickens fed a corn/soybean-diet without and with highly methylated citrus pectin (HMC) from 0 to 21 days of age.

| | Dietary treatment | | | |
	Maize	Maize +30g HMC/kg	SEM[1]	Sign. effect
Conventional chicks				
Body weight gain (g)	773	696	6.4	*
Food conversion ratio	1.33	1.54	0.008	*
Intestinal conditions				
Digesta viscosity (mPa.s)	1.7	60.8	0.35	*
Ileal pH	6.6	5.5	0.18	*
Rel. wt. small intestine (% BW)	6.6	8.8	0.13	*
Digestibility of				
Dry matter (%)	71.6	64.8	0.25	*
Fat (%)	81.3	65.7	0.66	*
Germ-free chicks				
Production performance				
Body weight gain (g)	737	694	11.2	*
Food conversion ratio	1.32	1.36	0.012	NS
Intestinal conditions				
Digesta viscosity (mPa.s)	2.2	7.3	0.39	*
Ileal pH	7.9	7.8	0.03	NS
Rel. wt. small intestine (% BW)	4.9	5.3	0.23	NS
Digestibility of				
Dry matter (%)	74.4	74.6	0.70	NS
Fat (%)	93.9	94.8	0.32	NS

[1] SEM value and significancies (NS: non significant; *: $P<0.05$) were based on three dietary treatments for production performances and intestinal conditions (Langhout, 1998), while only two are presented in this table.

system activation, which was realised via variation in weaning age, vaccination scheme, use of dietary antimicrobials and housing system. Results are summarised in Table 9. A high level of immune system stimulation resulted in a reduced feed intake, and daily gain (40% reduction of protein accretion, while fat deposition was not affected). This effect was probably due to a higher level of cytokine release as part of the immune response, which reduces protein accretion due to the synthesis of acute phase proteins in the liver.

Table 9. The impact of level of chronic immune system (IS) activation on efficiency and composition of growth in pigs fed from 6 to 27 kg body weight.

	IS activation	
	low	high
Growth and feed utilisation		
daily gain, g	973	863
feed to gain	1.44	1.81
Composition of body growth at 27 kg		
protein gain, g/day	105	65
fat gain, g/day	67	63

An immune stimulation affects protein and amino acid requirements. Several model calculations have been made to quantify nutrient costs for immune and inflammatory responses. If changes in the nutrient requirements of immune compromised animals are known, modifications in dietary nutrient composition might help to reduce production losses as indicated in Table 9.

Effects of immune stimulation on nutrient requirements of pigs can also be quantified using an in vivo model via an insulin infusion to modify the balance between anabolic and catabolic processes. Under normal physiological conditions insulin is secreted after a meal by the pancreas to ensure effective use of nutrients for anabolic processes. Insulin increases glucose-uptake, storage and oxidation; increases amino acid uptake and storage but decreases amino acid oxidation (and decreases gluconeogenesis from amino acids in the liver); decreases lipolysis and free fatty acid oxidation and increases de novo lipogenesis from glucose. The principle of this technique is that the animal's metabolism is switched on with an intravenous insulin-infusion in the absence of a meal. Due to the action of insulin, the animal will reveal its specific nutrient need related to age, gender and infection status. The amount of glucose or amino acid infused into the portal vein, necessary to maintain a constant nutrient level in the blood (on line measurements), is a direct reflection of the net metabolic use by the body (Figure 7). The net infusion of amino acids during insulin infusion are primarily used for net protein accretion, which will be muscle protein in healthy animals or used for liver metabolism in case of immune stimulated animals (for instance via a microbial challenge or a LPS injection).

As with glucose, the same principle applies for amino acids. For each individual amino acid, the net metabolic use can be measured by quantifying the portal amino acid infusion rate. Recently, the effect of a Salmonella enteritis challenge on the amino acid requirements was shown in a pilot study with growing pigs using the insulin clamp method. The lysine requirement was reduced by 50%, while the glutamine and tryptophane requirements were doubled and tripled respectively (Koopmans, personal communication). These effects were in line with effects hypothesised by Yoo et al (1997) for glutamine, by Klasing and Calvert (1999) for tryptophane, and by Stahly

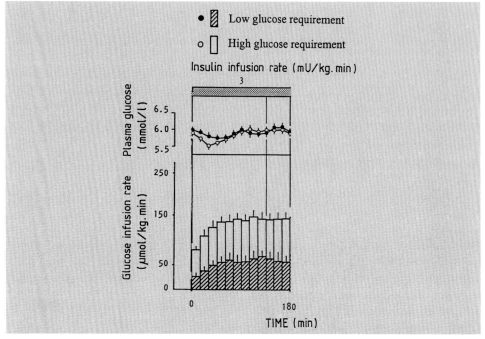

Figure 7. The net metabolic use of glucose at the whole body level. The example shows a group of pigs with low glucose utilisation and a group with high glucose utilisation. After initiation of the insulin infusion, it takes about 60-90 minutes to reach a stable (steady state) activation of metabolism. The last hour of the insulin infusion test is used to quantify net metabolic use of glucose.

(1996) for lysine but the magnitude of these effects can now be quantified. Such knowledge will be useful to formulate diets for (sub)clinically infected animals.

1.8. Concluding remarks

In this paper dietary effects on gut-health related parameters have been shown. Research models are available to study effects of gastro-intestinal stressors (like malnutrition of enterocytes directly after weaning of piglets and an increased microbial activity in the gastrointestinal tract of broilers) on the intestinal barrier function. It has been shown that digestion and absorption of nutrients from the small intestine are reduced and intestinal digestion is compromised by increased intraluminal microbial activities in broilers. Data with piglets suggest that an increased permeability of the intestinal mucosa is related to an inflammatory response, initiated by feed deprivation after weaning. Finally, nutrient expenditure in case of e.g. an inflammatory response can be quantified.

However, experiments carried out to correlate response parameters are scarce. Such experiments will help to better understand the cascade of reactions leading to a compromised gut health/gut integrity, and thereby in nutritional measures to counteract. These results might be incorporated in a gut health index in which the effect of different response parameters can be balanced and used to predict or describe the intestinal health status. A gut health index should include different intestinal functions, like microbial activity (e.g. ATP content), nutrient digestion (e.g. fat digestibility being very sensitive for disturbances), enterocyte differention (e.g. brush border enzyme activities, and morphometry), and barrier function (permeability measurements and possibly also bacterial translocation).

As long as such data are lacking, nutritionists will aim for an optimised or maximised digestion and absorption of nutrients, more or less hoping that the intestinal barrier function will not be compromised. Balancing all three aspects of the intestinal function will definitely improve the efficiency of nutrient utilisation, however, is not yet a reality.

1.9. References

Allen, P.C. (1999). Effect of daily oral doses of L-arginine on coccidiosis infections in chickens. Poultry Science 78: 1506-1509

Bedford, M. (2000). Removal of antibiotic growth promotors from poultry diets: implications and strategies to minimise subsequent problems. World's Poultry Science Journal 56: 347-365.

Brenes, A., M. Smith, W. Guenter and R.R. Marquardt (1993). Effect of enzyme supplementation on the performance and digestive tract size of broiler chickens fed wheat and barley based diets. Poultry Science 72: 1731-1739

Carré, B., J. Gomez and A.M. Chagneau (1995). Contribution of oligosaccharides and polysaccharide digestion, and excreta losses of lactic acid and short chain fatty acids, to dietary metabolisable energy values in broiler chickens and adult cockerels. British Poultry Science 36: 611-629.

Dänicke, S. (2000). Effects of non-starch polysaccharides (NSP) and NSP-hydrolysing enzymes on nutrient utilisation in poultry and pigs. In: Proceedings of the 3rd European Symposium on Feed Enzymes, Noordwijkerhout, The Netherlands.

Drochner, W. (1993) Digestion of carbohydrates in the pig. Archives for Animal Nutrition 43: 95-116.

Elkin, R.G., K.V. Wood and L.R. Hagley (1990). Biliary bile acid profiles of domestic fowl as determined by high performance liquid chromatography and fast atom bombardment mass spectrometry. Comp. Biochem. Physiol. B96: 157-161.

Ganessunker, D., H.R. Gaskins, F.A. Zuckermann and S.M. Donovan (1999). Total parenteral nutrition alters molecular and cellular indices of intestinal inflammation in neonatal piglets. Journal of parenteral and enteral nutrition 23: 337-344.

Grala, W. (1998). Nitrogen utilisation in pigs as affected by dietary induced losses of ileal endogenous nitrogen. PhD thesis, Agricultural University Wageningen, The Netherlands.

Green, J. and T.F. Kellogg (1987). Bile acid concentrations in serum, bile, jejunal contents, and excreta of male broiler chicks during the first weeks posthatch. Poultry Science 66: 535-540.

Helander, A. et al. (1997). Microbial Pathogenesis 23:335-346.

Huisman, J. (1999). Prospects in gastrointestinal physiology in pigs and veal calves. In: Nutrition and gastrointestinal physiology -today and tomorrow- pp 85-103.

Hurwitz, S., A. Bar, M. Katz, D. Sklan and P. Budowski (1973). Absorption and secretion of fatty acids and bile acids in the intestine of the laying fowl. Journal of Nutrition 103: 543-547.

Huurne, A. ter, S. Jeurissen, F. Lewis, J.D. van der Klis, Z. Mroz and A. Rebel (2000). Parameters and techniques used to determine intestinal health as constituted by integrity, functionality, immunity and microflora. Report ID-Lelystad, July 2000.

Hylemond, P.B. (1985). Metabolism of bile acids in intestinal microflora. In: Sterols and bile acids: New comprehensive biochemistry 1985, H. Danielsen and J. Sjovall (Eds.), Elseviers Science Publishers, pp 331-343

Jamroz, D., J. Orda, A. Wiliczkiewicz and J. Skorupinska (1996). The apparent digestibility of structural carbohydrates and the intestine fermentation of different kinds of grains in three poultry species Wiener Tierärztliche Monatschrift 83: 210-218.

Jansman, A.J.M., G.M. Beelen, G. Derksen, N.P. Lenis, J. van der Meulen, R. van der Weij-Jongbloed (1998a). Invloed van rantsoensamenstelling op de schijnbare ileale verteerbaarheid van nutriënten en op fermentatie in het verteringskanaal van varkens. TNO rapport I 96-31003.

Jansman, A.J.M., G.M. Beelen, P. van Leeuwen, J. van der Meulen, J.G.M. Bakker (1998b). Invloed van fermentatie in het verteringskanaal op de portale flux van nutriënten bij varkens. TNO rapport I 97-31055b.

Jansman, A.J.M., L.J.G.M. Bongers and P. van Leeuwen (2001). Effect of fermentable components in the diet on the portal flux of glucose and volatile fatty acids in growing pigs. In: Proceedings of the 8th Symposium on digestive physiology of pigs. Uppsala, Sweden.

Jensen, B.B. (1999) Impact of feed composition and feed processing on the gastrointestinal ecosystem in pigs. In: Nutrition and gastrointestinal physiology -today and tomorrow- pp 43-56.

Juste, A., J.A. Fernande, and H. Jorgenson (1983). Response of bile flow, biliary lipids and bile acid pool in the pig to quantitative variations in dietary fat. J. Nutr. 113: 1671-1701.

Kelly, D., J.A. Smyth and K.J. McCracken (1991). Digestive development of the early-weaned pig. 2. Effect of feed intake on digestive enzyme activity during the immediate post-weaning period. British Journal of Nutrition 65: 181-188.

Kelly, D. (1994). Colostrum, growth factors and intestinal development in pigs. In: Proceedings of the VIth International Symposium on Digestive Physiology in Pigs, pp 151-166. EAAP Publication no. 80, Bad Doberan, Germany.

Klasing, K.C. and C.C. Calvert (1998). The care and feeding of an immune system: an analysis of lysine needs. In: Protein metabolism and nutrition, Aberdeen, United Kingdom, pp 253-264.

Klis, J.D. van der (1993). Physico-chemical chyme conditions and mineral absorption in broilers. PhD thesis, Agricultural University Wageningen, The Netherlands.

Klis, J.D. van der, D.J. Langhout and J. de Jong (1999). The effect of water-soluble non starch polysaccharides on the microbial composition and activity and intestinal morphology of broilers. TNO report V99.017.

Klis, J.D. van der and C.H.M. Versantvoort (1999). On the relationship between intestinal morphology and absorptive capacity in broilers. In: Proc. of the 12th European Symposium on Poultry Nutrition, Veldhoven, The Netherlands, pp163-165.

Krogdahl, A. and J.L. Sell (1989). Influence of age on lipase, amylase and protease activities in pancreatic tissue and intestinal contents of young turkeys. Poultry Science 68: 1561-1568.

Laplace, J.P. (1982). Gastric function in the pig. In: Digestive physiology in the Pig. 2nd International Seminar, pp 29-45.

Langhout, D.J. (1998). The role of the intestinal flora as affected by non-starch polysaccharides in broiler chicks. PhD thesis, Agricultural University Wageningen, The Netherlands.

Langhout, D.J., J.B. Schutte, P. van Leeuwen, J. Wiebenga and S. Tamminga (1999). Effect of dietary high- and low-methylated citrus pectin on activity of the ileal microflora and morphology of the small intestinal wall of broiler chicks. British Poultry Science 30: 340-347.

Lilja, C. (1983) A comparative study of postnatal growth and organ development in some species of birds. Growth 47: 317-339.

Madara, J.L., S. Nash, R. Moore and K. Atisook (1988). Structure and function of the intestinal epithelial barrier in health and disease. In: Gastrointestinal pathology (Eds. H. Goldman, H.D. Appelman and N. Kaufman), pp 306-324

Masclee, A., A. Tangerman, A. van Schaijk, E.W. van der Hoek and H.M. van Tongeren (1989). Unconjugated serum bile acids as a marker of small intestinal bacterial overgrowth. European Journal of Clinical Investigations 19: 384-389.

McCracken, B.A. , H.R. Gaskins, P.J. Ruwe Kaiser, K.C. Klasing and D.E. Jewell (1995). Diet-dependent and diet-independent metabolic responses underlie growth stasis of pigs at weaning. Journal of Nutrition 125: 2838-2845.

Michael, E. and E.D. Hodges (1973). Histochemical changes in the fowl small intestine associated with enhanced absorption after feed restriction. Histochemistry, 36: 39-49.

Muramatsu, T., S. Nakajima and J. Okumura (1994). Modification of energy metabolism by the presence of the gut microflora in the chicken. British Journal of Nutrition 71: 709-717.

Nabuurs, M (1991). Etiologic and pathogenic studies on postweaning diarrhoea. PhD thesis University of Utrecht.

Nitsan, Z., G. Ben-Aviaham, Z, Zoref and J. Nir (1991). Growth and development of digestive organs and some enzymes in broiler chickens after hatching. Br. Poultry Sci. 34: 523-532.

Noack, J., B. Kleessen, A. Lorenz, and M. Blaut (1996). The effect of alimentary polyamine depletion of germ-free and conventional rats. Nutritional Biochemistry 7: 560-566.

Noy, Y. and D. Sklan (1995). Digestion and absorption in the young chick. Poultry Sci. 74: 366-373.

Nyachotti, C.M., C.F.M. de Lange, B.W. McBride and H. Schulze (1997). Significance of endogenous gut nitrogen losses in the nutrition of growing pigs. a. review. Canadian Journal of Animal Science 77: 149-163.

Pierzynowski, S.G, B.R. Westrøm, J. Svedsen, L. Svedsen, and B.W. Karlsson (1995). Development and regulation of porcine pancreatic function. Int. J. Pancreatol. 18: 81-94.

Pluske, J.R., D.J. Hampson and I.H. Williams (1997). Factors influencing the structure and function of the small intestine in the weaned pig: a review. Livestock Production Science 51: 215-236.

Rozee, K.R., D. Cooper, K. Lam and J.W. Costerton (1982). Microbial flora of the mouse ileum mucous layer and epithelial surface. Applied Environmental Microbiology 43: 1451-1463.

Schneeman, B.O., B.D. Richter and L.R. Jacobs (1982) Response of dietary wheat bran in the exocrine pancreas and intestine of rats. Journal of Nutrition 120: 1179-1184.

Schulze, H. (1994) Endogenous ileal nitrogen losses in pigs - dietary factors. PhD thesis, Agricultural University Wageningen, The Netherlands.

Seidel, E.R., M.K. Haddox and L.R. Johnson (1985). Ileal mucosal growth during intraluminal infusion of ethylamine or putrescine. American Journal of Physiology 249: G434-438.

Simon, O. (2001). The influence of feed composition on protein metabolism in the gut. In: Gut environment of pigs. A. Piva, K.E. Bach Knudsen and J.E. Lindberg (Eds.), Nottigham University Press, pp 63-84.

Smits, C.H.M. (1996). Viscosity of dietary fibre in relation to lipid digestibility in broiler chickens. PhD thesis, Agricultural University Wageningen, The Netherlands.

Souffrant, W.B. (1991). Endogenous nitrogen losses during digestion in pigs. In: Digestive physiology in pigs. Proceedings of the Vth international symposium on digestive physiology in pigs, pp 147-166.

Spreeuwenberg, M.A.M., J.M.A.J. Verdonk, H.R. Gaskins and M.W.A. Verstegen (2001). Small intestinal epithelial barrier function is compromised in pigs with low feed intake at weaning. Journal of Nutrition 131: 1520-1527.

Stahly, Ph.D. (1996). Impact of immune system activation on growth and optimal dietary regiments in pigs. In: Recent advances in animal nutrition. P.C. Garnsworthy, J. Wiseman and W. Haresign (Eds.) Nottingham University Press, United Kingdom, pp 197-206.

Thomson, A.B.R. and J.M. Dietschy (1977) Derivation of the equation that describes the effects of unstirred water layers on the kinetic parameters of active transport processes in the intestine. Journal of Theoretical Biology 64: 277-294.

Tarvid, I., L.Ma. Cranwell and R. Vavala (1994). The early postnatal development of protein digestion in pigs. 1. Pancreatic enzymes. In: 6th international symposium on digestive physiology in pigs, Bad Doberan, Germany, pp 199-202.

Uni, Z., G. Zaiger and R. Reifer (1998). Vitamin A deficiency induces morphometric changes and decreased functionality in chicken small intestine. British Journal of Nutrition 80: 401-407.

Uni, Z., Y. Noy and D. Sklan (1999). Posthatch development of small intestinal function in the poult. Poultry Science 78: 215-222.

Verdonk, J.M.A.J., M.A.M. Spreeuwenberg, G.C.M. Bakker and M.W.A. Verstegen (1999). Nutrient intake level affects histology and permeability of the small intestine of newly weaned pigs. In: Proceedings of the 8th Symposium on digestive physiology of pigs. Uppsala, Sweden.

Wagner, D.D. and O.P. Thomas (1987). Influence of diets containing rye or pectin on the intestinal flora of chicks. Poultry Science 57: 971-975.

Weiser, M.M. (1973) Intestinal epithelial surface membrane glycoprotein synthesis. Journal of Biological Chemistry 248: 2536-2541.

Yoo, S.S., Field, C.J. and McBurney, M.I. (1997). Glutamine supplementation maintains intramuscular glutamine concentrations and normalises lymphocyte function in infected early-weaned pigs. J. Nutr. 127: 2253-2259.

2. Dietary strategies to influence the gastro-intestinal microflora of young animals, and its potential to improve intestinal health

J. Snel[1], H.J.M. Harmsen[2], P.W.J.J. van der Wielen[3] and B.A. Williams[4]
[1] *NIZO food research, Nutrition, P.O. Box 20, 6710 BA Ede, The Netherlands*
[2] *Department of Medical Microbiology, University of Groningen, Hanzeplein 1, 9713 GZ Groningen, The Netherlands*
[3] *Centre for Veterinary Public Health and Environmental Protection, Utrecht University, P.O. Box 80175, 3508 TD Utrecht, The Netherlands*
[4] *Animal Nutrition Group, Wageningen Institute of Animal Sciences (WIAS), Wageningen University, Marijkeweg 40, 6709 PG, Wageningen, The Netherlands*

2.1. Introduction

The gastro-intestinal microflora of man and animals comprises several hundred species and up to 10^{12} bacteria per gram colonic contents (Moore and Holdeman, 1974). The majority of these bacteria are strict anaerobes. Both the variety of species as well as the microbial numbers in the gut are determined by an array of complex factors, including the pH of the intestinal contents, intestinal motility, immune activity, and feed composition. However, due to this complexity, our understanding of the microflora and its interactions with the host is still limited.

2.1.1. importance of the microflora for health

Taking into account the enormous surface area of the intestinal tract and the numerous bacteria in the intestinal contents, it is not surprising that intestinal bacteria have an influence on the host. Indeed, a comparison of conventional and germfree animals (the latter being free of bacteria), revealed that the gastro-intestinal microflora is important for the normal development of gut morphology and functioning. Germ-free animals had an enlarged caecum, a thinner mucosa and shorter villi and crypts (Abrams, et al., 1963). There were also physiological abnormalities found in these animals: for example, intestinal motility was reduced (Abrams and Bishop, 1967), the body temperature was slightly decreased (Kluger, et al., 1990) and the intestinal immune system was poorly developed (Berg and Savage, 1975, Umesaki, et al., 1993). All those characteristics were quickly restored after addition of a normal microflora to germfree animals.

It is widely believed that some intestinal bacteria are beneficial to health whilst others may be harmful. Pathogenic bacteria can have their harmful effects either through mucosal invasion or production of toxins or both. In this respect, most attention has been given to the gram-negative species, including *Salmonella*, *Campylobacter* and *Escherichia coli*. Potentially health-promoting bacteria on the other hand, are thought to include mainly the lactic acid-producing bacteria such as members of the genera *Lactobacillus* and *Bifidobacterium*. Although addition of these bacterial strains frequently leads to health promoting effects, their contribution when present as part of the normal flora is usually unknown, since control animals with a microflora that lacks these bacteria are difficult to obtain. Of special interest are the segmented filamentous bacteria. These as yet unculturable bacteria adhere strongly to the epithelial cells of the ileum and Peyer's patches. As a result, they stimulate the intestinal immune system (Snel, et al., 1998). Furthermore, they prevent adhesion of other bacteria by competition (Heczko, et al., 2000), and possibly by alterations of the glycolipids on epithelial cells (Umesaki, et al., 1997). These bacteria have been found in many animal species including chickens (Allen, 1992), pigs (Sanford, 1991), cattle (Smith, 1997) and horses (Lowden and Heath, 1995). A schematic overview of the potential activities of beneficial bacterial cells in the intestinal tract is shown in Figure 1.

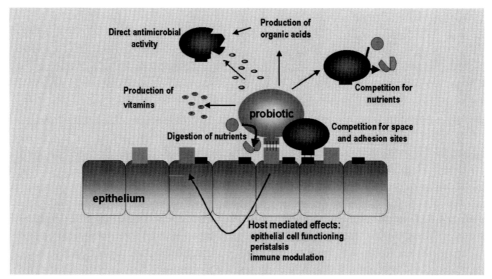

Figure 1. Schematic representation of the potential activities of a beneficial bacterial cell in the intestinal tract. Bacteria express activities towards other bacteria such as the production of antimicrobial components and competition for space and nutrients. Next to that, there is a strong interaction with epithelial cells resulting in an influence on the host physiology. The activities of a bacterium are strain-dependent.

2.1.2. Colonization and colonization resistance

The microflora consists of transient bacteria which only reside in the tract temporarily, and indigenous bacteria that permanently colonize the intestinal tract. Colonization by a bacterial species is defined as a bacterial population in the gastrointestinal tract which is stable in size and occurrence over time, without the need for periodic re-introduction of bacteria by repeated oral doses or other means. This implies that colonizing bacteria multiply in a particular intestinal niche, at a rate that equals or exceeds their rate of washout or elimination at the site (Mackie, et al., 1999). Therefore, association with the intestinal wall is likely to be an important factor for bacteria to maintain themselves at specific locations in the intestinal tract. The mechanisms by which the different bacteria adhere to the intestinal epithelium are largely unknown. An interesting observation with regard to colonization, is that certain species within the microflora can influence the expression of glycoconjugates on epithelial cells that may serve as receptors for adhesion of bacteria (Bry, et al., 1996, Umesaki, et al., 1997). In this way, they can influence colonization by other species. For example, *Bacteroides thetaiotaomicron* and segmented filamentous bacteria induce the fucosylation of the glycolipid asialo GM1 on epithelial cells of the small intestine in mice. As a result of this mutually beneficial "crosstalk" between the microflora and the host, these species are stimulated, whereas attachment of *Enterobacteriaceae* to epithelial cells is likely reduced (Umesaki, 1989) since these species prefer adhesion to asialo GM1 rather than to fucosyl asialo GM1. As a result, the presence of *Bacteroides* may reduce colonization of members of *Enterobacteriaceae* such as *E. coli* and *Salmonella*.

The indigenous microflora tends to suppress colonization of newly entering bacteria by a process called colonization resistance (Van der Waaij, et al., 1971). Even bacteria that are present in extremely low numbers can be important for colonization resistance. Germfree mice that were given a 1:1000 dilution or more of a normal microflora showed a disturbed colonization resistance (Koopman, et al., 1984). Decreased colonization resistance is frequently accompanied by overgrowth of pathogenic bacteria, leading to increased translocation of pathogens, and increased animal mortality. Part of the mechanism by which colonization resistance is thought to work is that the microbial ecosystem of the gut makes such efficient use of all available ecological niches that it remains very stable in terms of its composition. This stability limits both the availability of space and nutrients for newly entering species. The majority of the intestinal bacteria are strict anaerobes. Therefore an experiment was designed to investigate the combined effect of 95 anaerobic bacteria on *Shigella flexneri* levels in ex-germfree mice. Although *Shigella* levels were strongly reduced, a much better effect was observed if *E. coli* was administered in addition to the anaerobes, indicating that not only anaerobes but also aerobes are involved in colonization resistance (Freter and Abrams, 1972). Similar results were obtained in chickens: it was reported that a bacterial mixture of 295 strains of obligate anaerobic bacteria did not protect broilers which were subsequently infected with *Salmonella infantis* (Goren, et al., 1984a).

It can be concluded that both the individual bacterial species of the microflora and the microbial ecosystem in total, are important for intestinal health. This opens possibilities to develop strategies to determine whether or not the composition of the intestinal microflora can be improved. Successful strategies should contribute to the stability of the ecosystem or improve physiological functions such as immune reactivity and nutrient absorption. Also, dietary interventions could suppress the activities of (potentially) pathogenic bacteria, thereby preventing the detrimental effects of these microorganisms on intestinal wall integrity . Since the microflora of young animals is not stable in time, knowledge concerning the development of the microflora is of essential importance.

2.2. Development of the microflora

Microbial succession during the first few weeks of life in the alimentary tracts of humans, chicks, pigs, and calves is remarkably similar (Mackie, et al., 1999). Before birth or hatching, the intestinal tract is sterile (Kenworthy and Crabb, 1963). The young mammal encounters its first bacteria in the vagina of the mother, and then, after expulsion from the vagina, comes into contact with the large population of microbes present in both the faeces of its mother and within its new environment. By 5 - 6 hours after birth, the number of bacteria of the first colonizing species is already very high (10^9 to 10^{10} /g faeces). Colonization by bacteria occurs very rapidly and can be complete within two days. The rate of increase of bacteria can vary according to host species (Ewing and Cole, 1994).

In human babies, *Escherichia coli* and *Streptococcus* species rapidly colonize the intestinal tract of humans, followed by a sharp increase of *Bifidobacterium* species in breast-fed children. In contrast, formula-fed babies develop a more complex microflora with relatively high numbers of *Bacteroides*, *Clostridium* and *Streptococcus*, indicating the importance of the diet on microflora development (Harmsen, et al., 2000b). After weaning, the normal adult flora develops and remains stable.

2.2.1. Pigs

It appears that the newly born animal possesses a very efficient microbial selection system, since it seems to be able to modify the various bacterial ecosystems it encounters to produce relatively environmentally constant internal gut conditions. The first bacteria which become established in the digestive tract originate from the dam or the environment, but are not necessarily the most abundant ones within the ecosystems encountered by the young animal. For example, in a split litter experiment, five piglets were obtained aseptically and kept in a sterile cage. These aseptically "born" piglets had a similar population of microflora within the small intestine at one week, compared to those reared on the sow (Ducluzeau, 1985). There was a rapid establishment and implantation of *E. coli* and *Streptococcus* followed by *Lactobacillus* and *Clostridium*. However, even though clostridia were among the dominant species in the faeces or on the teats of the sow, they failed to become dominant in the gastro-intestinal tract of the piglets reared with their dam. It should be noted that these studies were probably carried out under conditions that did not allow the detection of non-sporulating strict anaerobes, and if repeated today might have detected a wider range of bacteria.

After this initial colonization, the bacterial population remains fairly stable during suckling, although qualitative changes do occur (Drasar and Barrow, 1985). However, the introduction of solid food causes major qualitative and quantitative alterations in microflora as the strict anaerobes such as *Bacteroides* gain ascendancy with a concomitant decline in levels of the facultative organisms (Savage, 1977). Hence, it has been realized that diet is important in the establishment of the gastro-intestinal microflora and that the diet of the suckling piglet is interesting. While it may be assumed generally that it comprises mainly sow's milk together with supplementary solid feed, piglets also consume considerable quantities of sow's faeces and bedding. The nature of the faeces, particularly in relation to any harmful micro-organisms, is therefore of great importance.

The extrinsic (environmental) and intrinsic (host) factors controlling which of the ingested bacteria will establish and the order of succession of the colonizing strains, is of major importance. However, this is a difficult topic to study because of the extreme subject variability, great variation in rearing and feeding practices, and limitations in sampling and analyzing gut microbial communities (Mackie, et al., 1999). Extrinsic factors of importance include the microbial load of the immediate environment, food and feeding habits, environmental temperature, and composition of the maternal microflora. Intrinsic factors include intestinal pH and redox potential, microbial interactions, physiological factors, peristalsis, bile acids, host secretions, immune responses, and bacterial mucosal receptors (Mackie, et al., 1999). Novel methods to analyse the microbial populations in the gut will be discussed in section 4 and 5.

2.2.2. Poultry

The main differences between modern poultry husbandry and modern farm mammal husbandry are the absence of a weaning period and a complete loss of contact with the mother in chickens. In the wild, newly hatched birds come into contact with faecal bacteria from the mother bird, which results in rapid development of the intestinal microflora. It is believed that lack of contact results in a delayed development of the intestinal microflora. In the first week of life, enterococci and lactobacilli dominate the crop, duodenum and ileum of broilers while coliforms, enterococci and lactobacilli dominate the caeca (Table 1) (Barnes, et al., 1972, Mead and Adams, 1975, Van der Wielen, et al., 2000). Thereafter, a complex microflora with mostly obligate anaerobic bacteria starts to dominate the caeca (Barnes, et al., 1972, Mead and Adams, 1975, Van der Wielen, et al., 2000), while lactobacilli dominate the crop, duodenum and ileum (Table 1) (Barnes, et al., 1972). After two to three weeks , the microflora is established in the intestine of broiler chickens, which is indicated by the stable bacterial fermentation products (lactate, propionate, acetate and butyrate) in the intestines. Lactate is the dominant fermentation product in the crop, duodenum and ileum, while acetate is only detectable in the crop at low concentrations (Table 2) (van der Wielen, unpublished results). In the caecum, acetate, propionate and butyrate are

Table 1. Bacterial numbers (log cfu g^{-1}) in different parts of the intestinal tract of broiler chickens (raised in a commercial farmhouse) at different ages. Values are given as the mean (standard deviation) of three chickens (van der Wielen, unpublished results).

	Crop			Ileum			Caecum		
	3-day-old	8-day-old	15-day-old	3-day-old	8-day-old	15-day-old	3-day-old	8-day-old	15-day-old
Enterobacteriaceae	5.7 (0.6)	5.7 (0.5)	4.6 (0.4)	4.9 (1.2)	7.4 (0.5)	6.1 (2.2)	9.4 (1.0)	7.7 (0.6)	8.7 (0.4)
Enterococcus	7.4 (0.2)	6.3 (0.7)	4.9 (0.6)	7.5 (0.4)	7.8 (0.6)	6.5 (1.6)	10.0 (0.1)	8.0 (0.2)	7.9 (0.6)
Lactobacillus	8.7 (0.3)	8.9 (0.5)	9.2 (0.1)	8.3 (0.1)	8.3 (0.4)	8.9 (0.2)	8.7 (1.0)	9.1 (0.2)	8.8 (0.4)
Total aerobic	8.5 (0.9)	8.6 (0.2)	8.9 (0.3)	8.4 (0.2)	8.7 (0.4)	8.9 (0.3)	10.0 (0.2)	8.7 (0.4)	9.0 (0.2)
Total anaerobic	8.7 (0.2)	8.6 (0.2)	8.9 (0.1)	8.5 (0.1)	8.7 (0.4)	8.7 (0.2)	10.0 (0.1)	9.3 (0.2)	9.9 (0.2)
Bacteroides	N.D.[a]	N.D.	N.D.	N.D.	N.D.	5.1 (1.5)	N.D.	4.0 (1.6)	7.6 (0.6)
Eubacterium	N.D.	N.D.	N.D.	N.D.	N.D.	N.D.	N.D.	N.D.	6.5 (0.6)

[a] means not detected.

Table 2. Concentrations of lactate, acetate, propionate and butyrate (μmol g-1) and pH levels in different parts of the intestinal tract of broiler chickens (raised in a commercial farmhouse) at different ages. Values are given as the mean (standard deviation) of three chickens (Van der Wielen, unpublished results).

	Crop		Ileum		Caecum	
	3-day-old	15-day-old	3-day-old	15-day-old	3-day-old	15-day-old
Lactate	94.8 (6.4)	114.5 (22.8)	22.5 (7.4)	47.5 (33.0)	12.1 (3.1)	20.2 (8.8)
Acetate	2.9 (0.0)	20.6 (13.7)	N.D.	1.4 (1.2)	17.4 (4.6)	72.9 (13.8)
Propionate	N.D.[a]	N.D.	N.D.	N.D.	N.D	6.9 (1.3)
Butyrate	N.D.	N.D.	N.D.	N.D.	N.D.	23.9 (10.5)
pH	4.7 (0.1)	5.0 (0.2)	7.3 (0.2)	6.7 (0.4)	5.8 (0.2)	5.8 (0.1)

[a] means not detected.

present in detectable amounts while lactate could only be detected in the first two weeks (Barnes, et al., 1979, Van der Wielen, et al., 2000). Recently, it has been shown that the undissociated form of volatile fatty acids is an important factor in reducing the number of *Enterobacteriaceae* and to a lesser extent enterococci during the development of the caecal microflora in broilers (Table 2) (Van der Wielen, et al., 2000). Although factors other than those already mentioned for mammals can also affect the development of the microflora in the intestinal tract of broiler chickens, the importance of these factors has not yet been evaluated thoroughly.

Dietary interventions which aim to improve the developing microflora frequently focus on the stability of the microflora during critical periods of an animal's life, i.e. immediately after birth or hatching, and in mammals during the weaning period. During these periods, the composition of the microflora changes dramatically and the diet may accelerate the development to a new stable ecosystem. Another target is the period shortly before slaughtering, since pathogens of the microflora may end up in the meat products. Other interventions, for example those that aim to improve feed conversion are not restricted to certain periods in the life of the growing animal.

2.3. Intervention: microflora management

Presently, there is a wide range of mainly dietary factors which affect the composition of the microflora. During intervention studies, any increase in bacterial numbers at a specific site in the intestinal tract is usually the result of outgrowth of bacteria that are already present at that site. The altered feed composition leads to new micro-ecological conditions that allows a better colonization of these species due to, for example, improved adhesion or growth rate. Alternatively, ingested bacterial species could potentially colonise the gastro-intestinal tract. This is the case when probiotics are administered to the animals. Microfloral management serves three purposes. Firstly, it may result in an improved feed conversion and weight gain. Secondly, microflora management can improve the intestinal health of the animals. Finally, these dietary interventions can suppress food-borne pathogens such as *Salmonella* and *Campylobacter* species. This is interesting for the production of meat and meat products that are safe for human consumption even when not thoroughly heated. The mechanisms by which the microflora is supposed to contribute to health are listed in Table 3.

Table 3. Mechanisms by which the microflora can contribute to intestinal health of animals and man.

Growth promotion
- improvement of the mucosal architecture
- degradation of unfermentable substrates into digestible components

Improvement of intestinal and general health
- breakdown of cytotoxic substances
- production of vitamins

Suppression of pathogens
- competition for nutrients
- competition for adhesion sites at the mucosal epithelium
- stimulation of intestinal motility
- stimulation of the immune system
- production of volatile fatty acids
- production of antimicrobial substances

All microfloral management strategies have in common that they aim to stimulate beneficial bacteria and suppress detrimental bacteria. This can be done by suppression of certain species as in the case of antibiotics and short chain fatty acids. Alternatively, beneficial species in the microflora can be promoted by feeding the animals suitable substrates such as oligosaccharides or other prebiotic fibres. In other cases, beneficial bacteria that are not present in the microflora can be added to the diet of the animals. Despite promising results in the development of new feed concepts to promote intestinal health, it should be noted that our knowledge concerning the interactions between bacteria in the gastrointestinal tract leading to a healthy microflora is still limited. This is complicated by the finding that the bacterial strains found in the gut vary from individual to individual (Kimura, et al., 1997, Zoetendal, et al., 1998). The current status of the most important intervention strategies is described in more detail below.

2.3.1. Antibiotics

Supplementation of animal feeds with sub-therapeutic levels of antibiotics has been used extensively in animal production, as it is purported to increase growth rate, especially in chickens and pigs. The exact mechanism by which anti-bacterial growth promoters exert their stimulatory effect is still unknown. However, (Yokoyama, et al., 1982) proposed that primary involvement of the gastrointestinal tract microflora could occur via the following possible mechanisms: 1) suppression of pathogens responsible for sub-clinical infections, 2) reduction of bacterial production of growth-depressing toxins, and 3) reduction of bacterial destruction and/or consumption of (essential) nutrients. This led to the suggestion that the stimulation of animal growth could be due to a beneficial shift in intestinal bacteria metabolism.

Exposure of animals to antibiotics, also exerts a selective pressure in the gastrointestinal environment which allows the proliferation of drug-resistant strains of bacteria, particularly *Enterococcus* (Barton, 2000). In most cases, the drug resistance is encoded on plasmids which may be transferred to other bacteria even in the absence of selection pressure by antibiotics. The implications of antibiotic-induced, transferable drug resistance in intestinal bacteria for human and animal health, and for treatment of disease are obvious and much discussed (Barton, 2000) and have led to restrictions on the use of anti-bacterial growth promoters in animal feeds (Mallett and Rowland, 1988).

The use of alternatives for antimicrobial growth promoters probably has economic consequences. This situation may change in the near future when the ban on growth promoting antibiotics in the EU is realised. Therefore, as our knowledge about the working mechanisms behind the alternatives is increasing, the use of these products may have a promising future for farm animal practice.

2.3.2. Probiotics

Already in 1907, it was proposed that consumption of live microorganisms (mainly lactic acid bacteria) could improve the intestinal health and well-being of the host (Metchnikoff, 1908, Metchnikoff, 1907). However, the actual term "probiotic" was first coined some three decades ago, although the meaning of the word has been changing ever since. Nowadays, a workable definition for probiotics is 'a mono- or mixed culture of live microorganisms which, when applied to animal or man, beneficially affect the host by improving the properties of the indigenous gastrointestinal micoflora' (Havenaar and Huis in 't Veld, 1992). Most probiotic research has been performed to improve the intestinal health of adult humans. *Lactobacillus rhamnosus* GG is one of the best-studied probiotics in humans and several studies have been done in relation to the health of infants. It was shown that strain GG can reduce (rotavirus-associated) diarrhoea in (premature) infants or newborns (Millar, et al., 1993, Sepp, et al., 1993). Furthermore, studies have shown an influence of this strain on the permeability of the intestinal barrier. It was observed that intake of this strain decreased the permeability for macromolecules and prevented the development of allergic reactions towards those macromolecules (Isolauri, et al., 1993).

In farm animals, the use of probiotics aims to improve intestinal health, which can then lead to a better general health and productivity. In young animals, the use of probiotics aims also to faster development of a stable intestinal microflora which, in turn, can improve the intestinal health of young animals. In piglets, several studies have shown a suppression of coliforms and clostridia in favour of lactic acid bacteria after treatment with probiotics during the weaning period (Mulder, et al., 1997, Nemcova, et al., 1999, Tortuero, et al., 1995). It was concluded from these studies that administration of lactic acid bacteria can result in a stabilized intestinal microflora during weaning and thereby improve the health status of the piglets.

Research in poultry has focused mainly on the selection of bacterial strains which reduce bacteria which are potential human pathogens such as *Salmonella* and *Campylobacter*. Infection with these bacteria does not usually result in clinical symptoms in poultry and pigs, although sometimes *Salmonella* can lead to disease in young broilers. Most reports on lactic acid bacteria did not show any protection against *Salmonella* (Adler and DaMassa, 1980, Opitz, et al., 1993, Soerjadi, et al., 1981) and some authors even suggested a negative effect of lactobacilli on intestinal balance, which can result in an increased colonization of *Salmonella* (Barnes, et al., 1980, Weinack, et al., 1985). Nevertheless, increased interest in the area of human probiotics has focused recent research once again on the use of lactobacilli as protective cultures against Salmonella. Some of these new studies show a protective effect of lactobacilli against *Salmonella* (Edens, et al., 1997, Pascual, et al., 1999) although the protection is much lower than is observed with mixed cultures of bacteria.

There are clear indications that probiotic bacteria can enhance growth of the host. This is of special interest since the use of growth-promoting antibiotics in animal feed is under debate and will soon be banned within the countries of the European Union (EU). Positive results with probiotics indicate a possible alternative to the use of antibiotics. Several *Lactobacillus* cultures show a positive effect on weight gain and feed conversion rates in broiler chickens (Abdulrahim, et al., 1999, Zulkifli, et al., 2000). For piglets, it was observed that administration of *L. acidophilus* (Pollmann, et al., 1980), propionibacteria (Mantere-Alhonen, 1995) or bifidobacteria (Abe, et al., 1995) resulted in a significant increased weight gain and decreased feed conversion compared to the control. These last authors also observed that the survival rate of piglets was significantly higher when a mixture of bifidobacteria replaced growth-promoting antibiotics. In summary, administration of probiotics to piglets and broiler chickens has been shown to increase weight gain and decrease feed conversion and may therefore be a good substitute for growth promoting antibiotics.

Most studies have focussed on the probiotic activity of living bacteria in the intestinal tract. It cannot be excluded that bacteria which are killed by the gastro-intestinal conditions can also contribute to animal health if their metabolites are present in the feed (Ouwehand and Salminen, 1998). Many lactic acid bacteria produce bacteriocins that have antimicrobial activity. Furthermore, their proteolytic activity can lead to the formation of bio-active peptides from dietary proteins, including peptides with an antimicrobial effect. It is likely that bacteriocins and other antimicrobial peptides, if resistant to proteolysis in the gut, can have a modulatory effect on the microflora.

Although experiments using probiotics have shown promising results in terms of an improvement in the intestinal health of farm animals, the use of probiotics in farm animal husbandry is not yet widespread. Research into the area of probiotics to improve the health status of pigs is relatively new. The exact working mechanisms are still largely unknown, and the bacterial strains which are presently in use could be easily replaced by improved strains in the near future.

2.3.3. Competitive exclusion

In poultry, the probiotic concept is usually referred to as 'competitive exclusion' although the working mechanisms are probably not essentially different. Usually a complex mixture of bacterial species is used rather than a single strain. Competitive exclusion has mainly been used to achieve a reduction of *Salmonella* serotypes that are pathogenic for humans rather than for the improvement of intestinal health of the bird itself.

Lack of contact between hatched chickens and the mother bird can result in a delayed development of the intestinal microflora in broiler chickens and subsequently a high susceptibility of young broilers to caecal *Salmonella* colonization. It was found that after administration of caecal material from an adult chicken to 1-day-old broilers, the animals had significantly lower counts of *Salmonella* in their caeca. (Nurmi and Rantale, 1973). Similar protection was observed when an anaerobic broth culture of caecal contents from adult fowl was used, whereas bovine rumen fluid and horse faecal material did not show any protective effect (Rantale and Nurmi, 1973). This work has been confirmed by many other research groups all over the world (reviewed by (Mead and Barrow, 1990)).

In the Netherlands, a big field trial was conducted with administration of undefined caecal cultures to one-day old broilers at the hatchery. The study included as many as eight million broilers in 284 flocks. Results showed that only 0.9% of the treated birds were Salmonella-positive compared to 3.5% of the control birds. Furthermore, competitive exclusion treatment reduced the *Salmonella*-incidence within positive flocks from 14.3% to 6.4% (Goren, et al., 1988, Goren, et al., 1984b). In spite of these successful results, the use of competitive exclusion cultures was stopped since most *Salmonella* serotypes found in broiler flocks had originated from their breeding farms of origin. Furthermore, the costs of treatment were high and the competitive exclusion product was undefined (Mulder and Bolder, 1991a). The main disadvantage of the undefined mixtures is the risk that they contain (potentially) pathogenic bacteria or viruses for poultry and/or humans, which makes it difficult to register undefined cultures in some countries and certainly within the European Union. Another consideration is that the mass production of well-defined mixtures of bacteria is much easier.

Therefore, attempts to develop a defined competitive exclusion culture have focused on mixtures of different known strains. It was observed that good protection against *Salmonella* infection was observed if the mixtures contained a large number of different bacterial strains (from 29 to 50 different strains) isolated from the caeca of adult chickens (Corrier, et al., 1995, Impey, et al., 1982, Stavric, et al., 1991). If the number of strains in these mixtures was reduced, the protection against *Salmonella* infection in broilers was much less pronounced (Corrier, et al., 1995, Nisbet, et al., 1993, Stavric, et al., 1991, Stavric, et al., 1985).

It was observed for competitive exclusion culture experiments that the decreased viable counts of Salmonella in caeca of 10-day-old treated broilers was negatively correlated with concentrations of (undissociated) volatile fatty acids in the caeca of broilers 2 days after treatment (3-day-old broilers) (Nisbet, et al., 1996, Ziprin, et al., 1990). However, these authors did not conclude that propionate or total volatile fatty acids had caused the reduction in Salmonella. It could be that propionate or total concentrations of volatile fatty acids are an indication that the caecal bacterial strains applied have become established in the caeca at 3 days of age but that these bacteria inhibit Salmonella by other mechanisms. Recently, it was observed that a rapid increase of volatile fatty acid concentrations was directly responsible for reduction of Salmonella enteritidis growing in a sequentially-fed batch culture, which mimics the caecal ecophysiology of broilers (Van der Wielen, et al., 2001). This information could be very useful in further selection of bacterial strains within defined mixtures.

Research in the field of competitive exclusion has led to the manufacture of a few commercially available competitive exclusion cultures. The bacterial composition of the Finnish product Broilact®is undefined, but it does have a limited number of chicken intestinal bacteria (Hirn, et al., 1992). Laboratory studies showed a significant reduction of Salmonella in caecal contents of chickens treated with Broilact® (Nuotio, et al., 1992, Salvat, et al., 1992). Field trials have confirmed these results in several countries. In Finland, Broilact® was used to treat 400 flocks and left 192 flocks untreated during a period of 3 years (1986 to 1988). After three years, only 6.5% of the treated flocks were Salmonella-positive compared to 21% of the untreated flocks (Hirn, et al., 1992). Similar results have been reported in Sweden and France (Palmu and Camelin, 1997, Wierup, et al., 1992). In 1992, more than 70% of all broilers were treated with Broilact® in Finland.

Competitive exclusion cultures have also been studied for any protective effect they may have against other enteropathogenic bacteria such as Campylobacter. The mixtures induced a reduction in the percentage of broilers shedding Campylobacter. However, a considerable number of birds were still Campylobacter positive in the treated group and therefore the protective effect would seem to be much lower than was observed for Salmonella (Hakkinen and Schneitz, 1999, Mead, et al., 1996, Mulder and Bolder, 1991b, Stern, 1994). However, some studies showed a very good protective effect against Campylobacter when broilers were treated with (un)defined competitive exclusion cultures (Schoeni and Wong, 1994, Soerjardi-Liem, et al., 1984). The protective effect of Broilact® against pathogenic E. coli has been described (Hakkinen and Schneitz, 1996), and it was shown that another competitive exclusion product induced protection against Listeria monocytogenes in leghorn chickens (Hume, et al., 1998).

Recently, the concept of competitive exclusion, in which a mixture of strains is used, has been extended to pigs and cattle. In pigs, an undefined competitive exclusion culture was isolated from the caecal mucosa of a healthy 6-week-old piglet (Fedorka-Cray, et al., 1999). When this culture was given to suckling pigs and these pigs were subsequently infected with Salmonella cholerasuis, a reduction of positive gut tissue

(28%) compared to the non-treated pigs (78%) was observed. The viable counts of *Salmonella* from caecal contents of treated pigs was 2-5 log lower compared to the non-treated group, indicating that competitive exclusion may also be useful in controlling *Salmonella* in young pigs (Fedorka-Cray, et al., 1999). Using another preparation of an undefined competitive exclusion culture, the same effect on *S. cholerasuis* was observed in pigs although no statistical analysis was done in that study (Anderson, et al., 1999). This competitive exclusion culture was also shown to reduce an enterotoxigenic *E. coli* infection in nursery-raised neonatal pigs (Genovese, et al., 2000). In cattle, a defined competitive exclusion culture of 17 strains of *E. coli* and 1 strain of *Proteus mirabilis* was administered to calves, which were infected with *E. coli* O157:H7 two days later. It was observed that the treated calves showed a reduced level of carriage of *E. coli* O157:H7 compared to the non-treated calves and it was therefore concluded that the use of these cultures might be a useful method to reduce the carriage of *E. coli* O157:H7 in cattle (Zhao, et al., 1998).

2.3.4. Prebiotics

Of the many factors which affect the composition of the large intestinal microflora, and the most influential in terms of microbial activity, is probably the type, amount and availability of growth substrate which is present at a particular site. Dietary residues which are undigested in the upper gastrointestinal tract, as well as endogenous material such as mucins, sloughed epithelial cells, and bacterial lysis products, contributes to the pool of available substrates (Collins and Gibson, 1999). Bacteria in the colon metabolize available carbohydrates to obtain energy for their own growth and maintenance (including motility, enzyme synthesis, maintenance of ionic and osmotic gradients, and active ion transport). One of the easiest ways to manipulate the residues which become available as substrates for the microflora, is by changes to the animal diet, such as by the addition of prebiotics. A "prebiotic" has been defined as a non-digestible food ingredient that beneficially affects the host by selectively stimulating the growth, activity or both, of one or a limited number of bacterial species already resident in the large intestine (Gibson and Roberfroid, 1995). Prebiotics have the advantage, compared with probiotics, that bacteria are stimulated which are normally present in the GIT of that individual animal and therefore already adapted to that environment.

The addition of prebiotics is increasingly being practised in both the food and feed industries. The potential beneficial effects of prebiotics have been summarized (Stewart et al., 1993) as being: antagonism towards pathogens, competition with pathogens, stimulation of enzyme reactions, decrease in ammonia and phenol production, and increased colonization resistance. Given that the amount and composition of substances reaching the large intestine can be readily modified by diet, it is probably the carbohydrate fraction (oligosaccharides, non-starch polysaccharides (NSP), and starches), which is most important in terms of bacterial substrates (Mathers and Annison, 1993). It is thought that the carbohydrate fraction can stimulate the growth of certain microorganisms, which produce VFA, and use ammonia as their source of nitrogen (Williams, et al., 2001). The ideal and most effective prebiotic would also be able to reduce or suppress the numbers and activities of known pathogens (Steer, et al., 2000). For example, some compounds have been shown to have specific effects on individual microbial species. Substances such as mannose (Ofek, et al., 1977), and galactan (Mathew, et al., 1993) have been found to block adherence of pathogenic *E.coli* strains, though the exact mechanism for this action is still poorly understood.

It has been shown that different carbohydrates can have very different rates of fermentation (Bauer et al., 2001) as well as variation in their production of end-products. This has been suggested to have important implications in terms of where the fermentation is most likely to take place in the GIT. For example, FOS, which is rapidly fermentable, has been shown to be completely fermentable prior to the terminal ileum of the pig (Houdijk, 1998), which means that it will not be available to provide energy for bacteria living in the caecum and colon. To stimulate fermentation in these areas, it would therefore be necessary to have a source of more slowly fermentable carbohydrate present in the diet (Williams B.A. *unpublished data*). The current status of prebiotics is that they alter the gut flora composition towards a purportedly healthier community. However, there are many other desirable attributes that could also be considered. Enhanced prebiotic properties which have been proposed (Steer, et al., 2000) include:

1. Highly selective fermentation; this would ensure stimulation of specific species of beneficial microorganisms, and more consistent production of end-products.
2. Increased persistence through the gastrointestinal tract; allowing fermentation of carbohydrate vs protein to take place along the entire GIT.
3. Anti-adhesive prebiotics; such as those found by Pusztai et al (1993) whereby lectins of snowdrop bulbs were shown to bind to mannose residues on epithelial cells, which are the adhesion sites for type 1 fimbriae of *E. coli*. This leads to a significantly reduced adhesion of pathogenic *E.coli*.
4. Attenuation of virulence of pathogens; the activity of pathogenic microorganisms can be strongly reduced by alterations in the intestinal environment. This is little investigated until now, but a promising possibility.
5. Reduction of gas production; leading to fewer cases of bloating and feelings of discomfort.

2.3.5. Organic acids

In poultry, it was observed in competitive exclusion studies that volatile fatty acids may be responsible for the observed reduction of *Salmonella* in the caeca of broiler chickens. Therefore, studies were conducted to determine the effect of addition of volatile fatty acids to the feed on *Salmonella* carriage in broilers. It was observed that feed treated with formic acid reduced the number of *Salmonella* positive caeca in a laboratory-scale experiment and in a small field trial (Hinton and Linton, 1988, Humphrey and Lanning, 1988). It remains uncertain from these studies if the formic acid reduces *Salmonella* in the intestines or in the feed, since the broilers were infected by adding *Salmonella* to the acid-treated feed. Studies in which propionic acid was added to the feed and chickens were orally infected, showed no reduction in *Salmonella* numbers from intestinal samples compared to the broilers receiving feed without propionic acid (Hume, et al., 1993a, Izat, et al., 1990). In contrast, others found that adding 1% formic or 1% propionic to the feed could significantly reduce the numbers of caecal *Salmonella*, but chickens were housed in individual isolators during this experiment, which may have affected the level of *Salmonella* infection (McHan and Shotts, 1992). Values for pH in different parts of the intestinal tract, weight gain or feed conversion were not affected by inclusion of volatile fatty acids in the feed (Hume, et al., 1993a, Izat, et al., 1990, Thompson and Hinton, 1997). Studies showed that the addition of volatile fatty acids to feed resulted in higher concentrations of these acids in the upper part of the intestinal tract (i.e. crop and gizzard) (Hume, et al., 1993a, Thompson and Hinton, 1997). The chemical fate of ^{14}C-propionic acid was followed in broilers fed with this radio-labelled propionate. Results showed that the label could only be detected in the foregut and not in the lower digestive tract or caeca (Hume, et al., 1993b). This is a very strong indication that addition of volatile fatty acids does not affect the intestinal microflora in the lower digestive tract of broilers.

2.3.6. Minerals

Dietary supplementation with high levels of minerals such as copper, zinc and calcium have received increasing interest in terms of their possible modulating effect on the microflora. In the intestinal tract, these minerals are only partly absorbed from the feed. Non-absorbed minerals could therefore interfere with biochemical processes that take place in the intestinal tract.

In piglets that received 2500 ppm zinc oxide in their diet, a decrease in the variety and diversity of coliforms was observed during the weaning period, although the total number of coliforms and enterococci was not reduced (Jensen-Waern, et al., 1998, Katouli, et al., 1999). It was concluded that supplementation with zinc oxide helped to maintain the stability of the intestinal microflora and might be beneficial in the prevention of post-weaning diarrhoea in pigs. Pigs and broilers that received 250 ppm copper sulphate in their diet have shown an improved weight gain and feed conversion (Hill, et al., 2000, Miles, et al., 1998). This effect might be related to copper-induced changes in the microbial composition comparable to the effects of zinc, though this has not been confirmed as yet. Although the effects of both copper sulphate and zinc oxide look promising, it should be realised that most of the minerals will not be absorbed by the animals and therefore end up in the environment. Here, they can affect ecosystems and therefore have to be considered as environmental pollutants. For this reason, the use of high levels of copper and zinc is restricted in several countries.

Recently, it was shown in rat studies that dietary calcium phosphate stimulates lactic acid bacteria that are present in the microflora. This resulted in an increased resistance towards a *Salmonella* infection in these animals: an increase in calcium from 0.8 g/kg to 7.2 g/kg resulted in a more than 100-fold reduction of salmonella excretion in faeces at day 3 of the infection (Bovee-Oudenhoven, et al., 1999). These authors further demonstrated that calcium acted to precipitate certain cytotoxic components within the intestinal lumen, such as bile salts and long-chain fatty acids, to which

Lactobacillus species have been shown to be extremely sensitive. Although the addition of rather high amounts of calcium seems to be common practice in the feed industry, there might be substantial differences in effect, depending upon the source of calcium used.

2.4. Tools for analysis of the microflora

Studies of the intestinal microflora have been hampered by a lack of methods to identify and enumerate the diversity of species in the intestinal tract. Conventional methods for determining the microfloral composition of the intestinal tract rely on the cultivation of bacteria onto anaerobic selective media. Although the introduction of anaerobic culture techniques led to a great improvement, there is still only a maximum of 20-40% of the intestinal bacteria which can be cultured. The reason for this is that many bacteria are difficult to culture or are unculturable due to a lack of suitable media (Ward, et al., 1992, Wilson and Blitchington, 1996). Quantification with culture techniques is not accurate since often media are not truly specific or are too selective for certain bacteria (Nelson and George, 1995). Furthermore, cultivation requires the immediate processing of samples which can be very labour-intensive.

To understand phenomena such as colonization resistance and immune stimulation, and to be able to evaluate the effect of treatments aimed at modulating the normal flora, it is important to have accurate means to enumerate and evaluate the various microbial populations. At present, most intervention studies aim to stimulate *Lactobacillus* and *Bifidobacterium* species. *E. coli*, as a representative of the *Enterobacteriaceae* family that is rich in pathogenic species, should be suppressed. There is still a need for new micro-ecological biomarkers that are indicative of an improved intestinal ecosystem. New molecular technologies have been developed that allow the analysis of microbial ecosystems, including the intestinal microflora, without the need for cultivation. It is expected that new biomarkers for intestinal health can be identified in studies in which these technologies have been used.

Molecular tools of modern microbial ecology have made it possible to study the composition of intestinal flora in a culture-independent way, mostly based on the detection of ribosomal RNA and DNA (rRNA and rDNA) (Amann, et al., 1995). Those tools are being increasingly used to determine the effects of dietary interventions on microfloral composition. The rRNA molecules have some characteristics which makes them particularly suitable as biomarkers. As part of the protein-synthesizing machinery of the cell, rRNA is present and has the same function in all organisms and can therefore be easily compared. The structure of the molecules is highly conserved, but contains enough variability to identify different bacteria to a species level. So far, mainly the 16S rRNA molecule has been used as a biomarker, because of its reasonable size of around 1500 base pairs and of the large extensive sequence information already available in the public databases such as the Ribosomal Database Project (RDP). The nine variable regions (V1 to V9) of the 16S rRNA molecule can serve as target site for detection of specific species or strains whereas more conserved areas allow detection of genera or groups of bacteria. For detection, specific oligonucleotides are used as primers in amplification techniques or as probes when labelled with a detectable molecule (e.g. fluorescent dye, radioactivity or an antigen). There are three techniques used extensively in microbial ecology, that are based on the variability in the 16S rRNA-gene (rDNA) or on the use of specific primers and probes based on 16S rRNA.

2.4.1. Fluorescent in situ hybridization (FISH)

With this technique, bacteria are stained fluorescently by hybridization with an rRNA-based oligonucleotide probe. For this, the bacteria need to be fixed with paraformaldehyde and/or ethanol, to maintain their morphology and to permeabilize their cell wall. Rigid cell walls of gram-positive bacteria may need extra enzymatic treatment. For instance, for faeces, different dilutions of a faecal suspension are applied to a glass slide and hybridized with a probe. After washing away the unbound probes, the slides are mounted and viewed with an epifluorescence microscope. By counting the number of bacteria per microscopic field which show fluorescence, and calculating the dilution factor of the original volume, quantitative results can be obtained (Franks, et al., 1998). The microscopic counting can be automated with a software driven microscope and image analyses (Jansen, et al., 1999). Quantitative results can also be obtained by hybridizing in suspension and analyzing the results by flow cytometry (Amann, et al., 1990).

2.4.2. Quantitative Polymerase Chain Reaction (Q-PCR)

With this technique, part of the microbial DNA is amplified using specific oligonucleotide primers. With PCR, a forward and reverse primer are attached to denatured target DNA and the primers are subsequently extended by a thermostable DNA-polymerase using a thermal cycler, thus copying the DNA strands between the primers. This cycle is repeated 30-40 times resulting in an exponential increase of this small piece of DNA. The amplification products are analysed afterwards on an ethidium bromide stained agarose gel where amplified DNA lights up as a band under UV light. Q-PCR is done on a real-time PCR machine with a built-in fluorimetric detection system for on-line quantification of amplification products. The formation of amplification products and the increase per cycle is then monitored while the process is running (real-time; see figure 2). The onset of the exponential phase of the curve showing the formation of amplification products is proportional to the amount of target DNA. In other words: the more target in the sample, the less cycles are needed for the amplification to become exponential. In this way, the amount of target DNA of a specific bacterium in a DNA sample, isolated from faeces or intestinal contents, can be quantified. Although a clear correlation of DNA quantification and colony forming units is observed, cell numbers cannot directly be calculated since the number of copies of the target gene depends on the growth phase and the number of target molecules per chromosome (Ludwig and Schleifer, 2000).

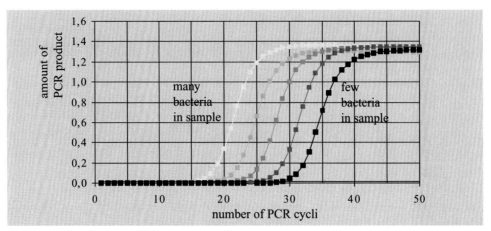

Figure 2. Typical profile of curves obtained using (quantitative) real-time PCR. During the PCR amplification process, oligonucleotide probes with both a reporter fluorescent dye and a quencher dye attached are degraded into smaller fragments. For the intact probe, the fluorescence is suppressed efficiently by the quencher dye due to its spatial proximity to the reporter. Therefore, the increase in reporter dye fluorescence is a direct consequence of target amplification. The use of a real-time PCR machine allows continuous monitoring of the fluorescence signal while the amplification proceeds. The amplification plot is dependent on the amount of target at the start of the PCR, and any inhibition of the amplification process can easily be monitored.

2.4.3. Denaturing Gradient Gel Electrophoresis (DGGE)

This technique is based on sequence-specific separation of 16S rDNA amplicons (Muyzer and Smalla, 1998). First, a variable part of the 16S rDNA is amplified by PCR with primers specific for all bacterial 16S rRNA (or rDNA). These amplicons are separated on a polyacrylamide gel containing a gradient of DNA-denaturing agents (urea/formamide) or on a temperature gradient. In this way, the amplicons are separated on the basis of their melting behaviour and GC content. When the DNA contains a large proportion of G and C nucleotides, the bonds between the DNA strands will be stronger, and the strands will denature at a higher concentration of denaturant than when lower levels of G and C are present. The sequence of nucleotides will also influence the melting behaviour of the strands. To keep strands together during electrophoresis, a 40-nucleotide stretch of G and C (GC-clamp) is attached to one of the primers. After electrophoresis the gel is stained, thus producing fingerprints of the community present within the sample. Individual amplicons (bands) can be identified by comparing those with PCR products of pure cultures or, by excising the band from the gel, re-amplifying it and analyzing its sequence.

In Table 4, the three techniques are compared showing their advantages and restrictions. Furthermore it gives a rough indication of the sensitivity of the methods, being estimations of the authors based on literature data. From this table, it can be concluded that the techniques complement each other and may be used in combination. Especially designing probes or primers on the basis of new sequences obtained by DGGE analysis and using them to quantify these organisms in the samples can make the approach complete. In this way any change in the total microflora can be studied in great detail.

Table 4. Advantages and restrictions of three molecular techniques for the quantification of bacteria in gastro-intestinal and faecal samples.

Advantages	Restrictions
DGGE	
Fingerprint of sample	Not quantitative
Unknown organisms can be analysed	Difficult to identify strains
Sensitivity: depends on specificity	RNA/DNA-isolation and PCR-amplification
Detection limits:	can cause biases
Non specific primers:	No morphological information
appr. 1% of population	
Group specific primers:	
$10^8 > x > 10^4$ bacteria/g faeces	
appr 10^{-3} % of population	
Q-PCR	
Quantitative	RNA/DNA-isolation can cause biases
High sensitivity	No morphological information
Detection limit:	Target must be known
$10^4 > x < 10^2$ CFU/g	
appr. 10^{-5}% of population	
Can be automated	
Fast	
FISH	
Quantitative	No physiological information.
Fast and inexpensive	Low sensitivity
Can provide distributional information	Detection limit:
Analysis by flow-cytometry or	$10^7 > x > 10^6$ bacteria /g of faeces
microscopic analysis which can be	appr. 10^{-2}% of population
automated	Target must be known
Gives morphological information	

2.5. Examples of some studies using molecular tools

Most studies on the composition of the intestinal microflora using molecular tools have been done using faecal samples. Especially in the case of human studies, this is usual for both practical and ethical reasons. However, it is questionable whether the faecal microflora is representative of the colonic microflora, since the gastro-intestinal content is very dynamic in its conversion from food to faeces. For the colonic microflora it is known that bacterial numbers increase during the passage through the colon, though the composition seems to remain stable (Finegold et al. 1983). Comparison of the faecal microflora composition with that of samples along the intestinal tract of pigs reveals clear differences (Simpson et al. 1999). In addition, a molecular cloning study of the bacterial microflora in different compartments of the gastrointestinal tract of pigs showed a clear difference between the bacterial composition of the colonic wall and the colonic and caecal lumen (Pryde et al. 1999). Therefore, although faecal samples may provide easily accessible samples, analysis of the dynamics of the colonic microflora requires the study of other samples, such as biopsies or material from sacrificed animals. Such samples are also needed to answer questions about other parts of the gastrointestinal tract.

One of the first papers to report the use of using gradient gel electrophoresis for studies in the gastrointestinal tract was by Zoetendal et al. (1998). They studied the diversity of the predominant bacteria in the human gastrointestinal tract. PCR amplicons of the V6 to V8 regions of faecal 16S rDNA were analyzed by temperature gradient gel electrophoresis (TGGE), a variant of DGGE. TGGE analysis of faeces from 16 individuals showed different profiles, with some bands in common. Faecal samples from two individuals were monitored over time and showed remarkably stable profiles over a period of at least six months. They combined the TGGE analyses with cloning and sequencing of the amplicons, and concluded that this combination is a reliable approach to monitor different microbial communities in faeces. In this paper, the investigators also showed that individual members of the community, represented as bands on the gels, could be identified by excising the bands from the gel and subsequently re-amplifying them and then sequencing . Furthermore, using simultaneous cloning strategies or PCR-amplification of pure cultures, marker samples can be constructed, which can be compared with the banding patterns, for a presumptive identification of the bands. In this line of research, Satokari et al. (2001) developed a DGGE-assay for human faeces with a primer set for a specific group of micro-organisms, i.e. *Bifidobacteria*. This was done to increase the sensitivity of this technique, and to be able to investigate specific sub-populations. This concept can easily be adapted for *Enterobacteriaceae* to study sub-populations such as *Escherichia* and *Salmonella*.

Simpson et al. (1999) investigated whether DGGE could be effectively applied to measure changes in bacterial populations of the pig gastro-intestinal tract, as influenced by age, diet or location. They analyzed the V3 region of 16S rDNA PCR products (approximately 200 bp) obtained from primers specific for the domain Bacteria. For this, they developed a protocol which included optimization of DNA extraction procedures, PCR amplification, removal of PCR artefacts, optimization of gel preparation and image capture. DGGE analysis revealed diverse bacterial populations between pigs of different ages and among individual gut compartments. Comparison of faecal DNA from pigs of different ages revealed several unique PCR product bands indicating the presence of unique bacterial populations. By comparing different gut compartments, they demonstrated that bacterial populations were most similar (C, value > 50%) within a single compartment and between adjacent ones. They concluded that DGGE can be used to examine bacterial diversity and population shifts in the pig gut. This is of special interest during the developmental period from birth through weaning, when the intestinal microflora undergoes a rapid ecological succession.

Q-PCR has only become available recently, but the developments in this field are very rapid. It is probably one of the most promising techniques when it comes to microbial diagnostics. However, applications in intestinal microbiology are still rare. Snel et al. (2000) used it to detect lactobacilli and *Salmonella* in faeces of rats that were fed different prebiotics, and subsequently infected with *Salmonella enteritidis*. Others have reported the use of Q-PCR to detect a numerically important anaerobic bacterium *Collinsella aerofaciens* in human faeces (Kageyama, et al., 2000). Identification of this species using culture techniques is very difficult and requires considerable time. Their Q-PCR system used *C. aerofaciens*-specific primers and a LightCycler1real-time PCR machine. Their assay used a double-stranded DNA dye to continuously monitor product formation and in a short time they were able to quantify samples to 5 log units in concentration.

Creelan and McCullough (2000) used Q-PCR to detect a strain-specific helicase gene of an ovine abortifacient strain (S26/3) of *Chlamydophila abortus (Chlamydia psittaci)* for the diagnosis of enzootic abortion in ewes (EAE). *C. abortus* DNA was amplified from tissues submitted from ovine abortion cases using strain-specific primers in a microvolume fluorimeter-based thermal cycler (LightCycler1). In this study, they compared Q-PCR with conventional PCR and with the standard of McCoy cell culture isolation. They concluded that it is a fast, sensitive, and specific method for the detection of EAE.

FISH using specific 16S rRNA-based oligonucleotide probes has been used to quantify bifidobacteria, lactobacilli and many other anaerobic bacteria in the human gut (Franks, et al., 1998, Harmsen, et al., 2000a, Harmsen, et al., 2000b, Langendijk, et al., 1995). It has also been used for the detection of salmonella in the mouse gut (Licht, et al., 1996). Specific oligonucleotide probes and primers have been designed, directed at different phylogenetic levels (domain, family, genus, species). They were designed for many bacterial species which are known to be present in the intestinal tract (Harmsen, et al., 2000a, Harmsen, et al., 2000b, Lin, et al., 1997, Sghir, et al., 1998, Simmering, et al., 1999), even for those that were hitherto non-culturable (Wilson and Blitchington, 1996). This list is still expanding rapidly.

In a study of Harmsen et al. (2000b) comparing breast-fed and formula-fed newborn infants, FISH with group-specific probes was used to analyze faecal samples without further culturing. Their results showed that FISH could be used to demonstrate the clear differences between the two groups both in development and in species diversity. The faeces of breast-fed babies contained more than 60% bifidobacteria while the faeces of formula-fed babies also contained many other species, such as *Bacteroides* and *E. coli*.

A combination of FISH, DGGE and culturing was applied in a study by Tannock et al. (2000). They monitored 10 healthy subjects before (6-month control period), during (6-month test period), and after (3-month post-test period) the administration of a milk product containing *Lactobacillus rhamnosus* DR20. Monthly faecal samples were examined by a variety of methods, including bacteriological culture analysis, FISH with group-specific probes and DGGE of the V2-V3 region of 16S rDNA amplicons. The composition of the cultured Lactobacillus population of each subject was analyzed by pulsed-field gel electrophoresis and by sequencing to the species level. The probiotic strain DR20 was detected in the faeces of all of the subjects during the test period, but at different frequencies. DR20 did not persist at levels of $>10^2$ cells per g in the faeces of most of the subjects after consumption of the product ceased. They concluded that consumption of the DR20-containing milk product transiently altered the Lactobacillus and enterococcal contents of the faeces of the majority of consumers without markedly affecting other bacteriological factors. DGGE and FISH analyses were mainly used to show that the other bacterial populations did not change due to the administration of the probiotic.

2.6. Other methods to study microflora

Instead of counting microorganisms, the magnitude of a whole mixed microbial population can also be determined by measuring microbial activity (Clarke, 1977). A measure of microbial activity may be obtained from production rates of microbial protein or fermentation end-products, or from turnover rates of various chemical pools that involve the microbes. When studying metabolism of the whole gut microflora, information on the metabolic reactions performed by the individual species comprising the flora is often of little use, since the colonic microflora of mammals is a very complex ecosystem of over 400 known microbial species, all of which can potentially interact and influence each other. Details of the metabolism of these species in terms of available nutrients are not known. Even if they were, it would be difficult to predict whether a reaction that occurs with a pure culture *in vitro* would also occur when the organism is interacting with other species *in vivo* (Rowland, 1992). The cumulative gas production method involves measurement of accumulating gas during fermentation, so that one obtains a picture of the kinetics of microbial activity of the population acting as a whole. At the end of the fermentation period, samples are taken for the measurement of VFA and ammonia, and for substrate utilization. Figure 3 gives an example of the kind of results one might obtain. In this case, piglets were fed either a control diet or a diet containing 10% sugar beet pulp. After 13 days on the diet, faeces was collected, and tested for its fermentation activity for sugar beet pulp *in vitro*. The technique was carried out under strictly anaerobic conditions, and was used to examine the activity of the microflora from many different sources, including different sections of the gastrointestinal tract of pigs (Williams, et al., 1997a), and the caeca of poultry (Williams, et al., 1997b). By using different starting substrates, it becomes possible to look at shifts in microbial populations which are associated with the fermentation of a particular feedstuff e.g. resistant starch, protein, or fibre (Williams, et al., 2000a).

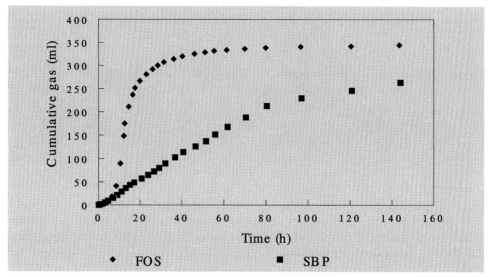

Figure 3. In vitro fermentation kinetics of sugar beet pulp (SBP) and fructo-oligosaccharides (FOS) using the same pig faeces as an inoculum.

Gibson and Fuller (Gibson and Fuller, 2000) described principles which were important for the development of both *in vitro* and *in vivo* techniques to identify probiotics and prebiotics as potential food additives. According to these principles, the cumulative gas production technique can also be used to test a range of different feed ingredients (or potential prebiotics) in order to assess the end-products of *in vitro* fermentation (Bauer, et al., 2001, Williams, et al., 2000b). Figure 4 shows the difference in fermentation kinetics between sugarbeet pulp and FOS using a single inoculum. While such a comparatively simple test can give a qualitative indication of the end-products that may be found *in vivo*, further research is needed to determine what the quantitative relations may be.

2.7. Conclusions

The microflora plays an important role in maintaining intestinal health and in the prevention of disease. One interesting possibility for the replacement of antibiotics as growth promoters for animal production, involves changes in the animal diet, which will stimulate the development of the autochthonous microflora of the host animal. Our increasing knowledge of the microfloral function allows the development of dietary strategies to shift the balance of the microbial ecosystem in a beneficial

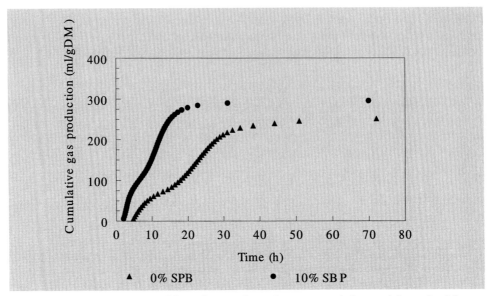

Figure 4. A comparison of faecal inoculum from two piglets, with and without sugarbeet pulp in the diet (0 and 10%) in terms of its activity (cumulative gas production) to ferment sugarbeet pulp in vitro.

direction. Some of these strategies have been validated and form attractive ways to improve intestinal health. Many of the proposed mechanisms still have to be evaluated in the near future. New tools to monitor the composition of the microflora form a valuable contribution to our present knowledge since many of the intestinal bacteria cannot be cultured and enumerated *in vitro*.

2.8. References

Abdulrahim, S.M., M.S. Haddadin, N.H. Odetallah, and R.K. Robinson. 1999. Effect of Lactobacillus acidophilus and zinc bacitracin as dietary additives for broiler chickens. British Poultry Science 40, 91-94.

Abe, F., N. Ishibashi, and S. Shimamura. 1995. Effect of administration of Bifidobacteria and lactic acid bacteria to newborn calves and piglets. Journal of Dairy Science 78, 2838-2846.

Abrams, G.D., H. Bauer, and H. Sprinz. 1963. Influence of the normal flora on mucosal morphology and cellular renewal in the ileum. Laboratory Investigations 121, 355-364.

Abrams, G.D., and J.E. Bishop. 1967. Effect of the normal microbial flora on gastrointestinal motility. Proceedings of the Society for Experimental Biology and Medicine 126, 301-304.

Adler, H.E., and A.J. DaMassa. 1980. Effect of ingested lactobacilli on *Salmonella infantis* and *Escherichia coli* and on intestinal flora, pasted vents, and chick growth. Avian Diseases 24, 868-878.

Allen, P.C. 1992. Comparative study of long, segmented, filamentous organisms in chickens and mice. Laboratory Animal Science 42, 542-547.

Amann, R.I., B.J. Binder, R.J. Olson, S.W. Chisholm, R. Devereux, and D.A. Stahl. 1990. Combination of 16S rRNA-targeted oligonucleotide probes with flow cytometry for analyzing mixed microbial populations. Applied & Environmental Microbiology 56, 1919-1925.

Amann, R.I., W. Ludwig, and K.H. Schleifer. 1995. Phylogenetic identification and in situ detection of individual microbial cells without cultivation. Microbiology Reviews 59, 143-169.

Anderson, R.C., L.H. Stanker, C.R. Young, S.A. Buckley, K.J. Genovese, R.B. Harvey, J.R. DeLoach, N.K. Keith, and D.J. Nisbet. 1999. Effect of competitive exclusion treatment on colonization of early-weaned pigs by Salmonella serovar Choleraesuis. Swine Health and Production 7, 155-160.

Barnes, E.M., G.C. Mead, D.A. Barnum, and E.G. Harry. 1972. The intestinal flora of the chicken in the period 2 to 6 weeks of age, with particular reference to the anaerobic bacteria. British Poultry Science 13, 311-326.

Barnes, E.M., C.S. Impey, and B.J. H. Stevens. 1979. Factors affecting the incidence and anti-salmonella activity of the anaerobic caecal flora of the young chick. Journal of Hygiene (Cambridge) 82, 263-283.

Barnes, E.M., C.S. Impey, and D.M. Cooper. 1980. Competitive exclusion of salmonellas from the newly hatched chicks. The Veterinary Record 106, 61.

Barton, M.D. 2000. Antibiotic use in animal feed and its impact on human health. Nutrition Research Reviews 13, 279-299.

Bauer E., B.A Williams, C. Voigt, R. Mosenthin, & M. Verstegen (2001) Microbial activities of faeces from unweaned and adult pigs, in relation to selected fermentable carbohydrates. Animal Science *accepted.*

Bauer, E., B.A. Williams, C. Voigt, R. Mosenthin, and M.W.A. Verstegen. 2001. A comparison of the fermentability of carbohydrate-rich feedstuffs, with and without enzyme pre-treatment. Animal Feed Science & Technology, submitted for publication.

Berg, R.D., and D.C. Savage. 1975. Immune responses of specific pathogen-free and gnotobiotic mice to antigens of indigenous and nonindigenous microorganisms. Infection & Immunity 11, 320-329.

Bovee-Oudenhoven, I.M., M.L. Wissink, J.T. Wouters, and R. Van der Meer. 1999. Dietary calcium phosphate stimulates intestinal lactobacilli and decreases the severity of a salmonella infection in rats. Journal of Nutrition 129, 607-612.

Bry, L., P.G. Falk, T. Midtvedt, and J.I. Gordon. 1996. A model of host-microbial interactions in an open mammalian ecosystem. Science 273, 1380-1383.

Clarke, R.T.J. 1977. Methods for studying gut microbes., p. 1-333. *In* R. J. Clarke and T. Bauchop (ed.), Microbial Ecology of the Gut. Academic Press, London.

Collins, M.D., and G.R. Gibson. 1999. Probiotics, prebiotics, and synbiotics: approaches for modulating the microbial ecology of the gut. American Journal of Clinical Nutrition 69, 1052S-1057S.

Corrier, D.E., D.J. Nisbet, C.M. Scanlan, A.G. Hollister, and J.R. DeLoach. 1995. Control of *Salmonella typhimurium* colonization in broiler chicks with a continuous-flow characterized mixed culture of caecal bacteria. Poultry Science 74, 916-924.

Creelan, J.L., and S.J. McCullough. 2000. Evaluation of strain-specific primer sequences from an abortifacient strain of ovine Chlamydophila abortus (Chalmydia psittaci) for the detection of EAE by PCR. FEMS Microbiology Letters 190, 103-108.

Drasar, B.S., and P. Barrow. 1985. Intestinal microbiology, vol. 10. American Society for Microbiology.

Ducluzeau, R. 1985. Implantation and development of the gut microflora in the newborn piglet. Pig News and Information 6, 415-418.

Edens, F.W., C.R. Parkhurst, I.A. Casas, and W.J. Dobrogosz. 1997. Principles of *ex ovo* competitive exclusion and *in ovo* administration of *Lactobacillus reuteri*. Poultry Science 76, 179-196.

Ewing, W.N., and D.J.A. Cole. 1994. The Living Gut: An Introduction to Micro-organisms in Nutrition. Context, Dungannon.

Fedorka-Cray, P.J., J.S. Bailey, N.J. Stern, N.A. Cox, S.R. Ladely, and M. Musgrove. 1999. Mucosal competitive exclusion to reduce Salmonella in swine. Journal of Food Protection 62, 1376-1380.

Finegold, S.M., V.L. Sutter, and G.E. Mathisen. 1983. Normal indigenous intestinal flora, p. 3-31. In D. J. Hentges (ed.), Human intestinal microflora in health and disease. Academic Press, New York.

Franks, A.H., H.J. M. Harmsen, G.C. Raangs, G.J. Jansen, F. Schut, and G.W. Welling. 1998. Variations of bacterial populations in human feces measured by fluorescent In situ hybridization with group-specific 16S rRNA-targeted oligonucleotide probes. Applied & Environmental Microbiology 64, 3336-3345.

Freter, R., and G.D. Abrams. 1972. Function of various intestinal bacteria in converting germfree mice to the normal state. Infection & Immunity 6, 119-26.

Genovese, K.J., R.C. Anderson, R.B. Harvey, and D.J. Nisbet. 2000. Competitive exclusion treatment reduces the mortality and faecal shedding associated with enterotoxigenic Escherichia coli infection in nursery-raised neonatal pigs. Canadian Journal of Veterinary Research 64, 204-207.

Gibson, G.R., and M.B. Roberfroid. 1995. Dietary modulation of the human colonic microbiota: introducing the concept of prebiotics. Journal of Nutrition 125, 1401-1412.

Gibson, G.R., and R. Fuller. 2000. Aspects of in vitro and in vivo research approaches directed toward identifying probiotics and prebiotics for human use. Journal of Nutrition 130, 391S-395S.

Goren, E., W.A. De Jong, P. Doornenbal, J.P. Koopman, and H.M. Kennis. 1984a. Protection of chicks against *Salmonella infantis* infection induced by strict anaerobically cultured intestinal microflora. The Veterinary Quarterly 6, 22-26.

Goren, E., W.A. De Jong, P. Doornenbal, J.P. Koopman, and H.M. Kennis. 1984b. Protection of chicks against salmonella infection induced by spray application of intestinal microflora in the hatchery. The Veterinary Quarterly 6, 73-79.

Goren, E., W.A. De Jong, P. Doornenbal, N.M. Bolder, R.W.A.W. Mulder, and A. Jansen. 1988. Reduction of salmonella infection of broilers by spray application of intestinal microflora: A longitudinal study. The Veterinary Quarterly 10, 249-255.

Hakkinen, M., and C. Schneitz. 1996. Efficacy of a commercial competitive exclusion product against a chicken pathogenic Escherichia coli and E. coli O157:H7. Veterinary Record 139, 139-141.

Hakkinen, M., and C. Schneitz. 1999. Efficacy of a commercial competitive exclusion product against Campylobacter jejuni. British Poultry Science 40, 619-621.

Harmsen, H.J., A.C. Wildeboer-Veloo, J. Grijpstra, J. Knol, J.E. Degener, and G.W. Welling. 2000a. Development of 16S rRNA-based probes for the coriobacterium group and the atopobium cluster and their application for enumeration of coriobacteriaceae in human feces from volunteers of different age groups. Applied & Environmental Microbiology 66, 4523-4527.

Harmsen, H.J., A.C. Wildeboer-Veloo, G.C. Raangs, A.A. Wagendorp, N. Klijn, J.G. Bindels, and G.W. Welling. 2000b. Analysis of intestinal flora development in breast-fed and formula-fed infants by using molecular identification and detection methods. Journal of Pediatric Gastroenterology & Nutrition 30, 61-67.

Havenaar, R., and J.H.J. Huis in 't Veld. 1992. Probiotics, a general view., p. 151-170. In B.J.B. Wood (ed.), The Lactic Acid Bacteria in Health and Disease., vol. 1. Elsevier, New York.

Heczko, U., A. Abe, and B.B. Finlay. 2000. Segmented filamentous bacteria prevent colonization of enteropathogenic Escherichia coli O103 in rabbits. Journal of Infectious Diseases 181, 1027-1033.

Hill, G.M., G.L. Cromwell, T.D. Crenshaw, C.R. Dove, R.C. Ewan, D.A. Knabe, A.J. Lewis, G.W. Libal, D.C. Mahan, G.C. Shurson, L.L. Southern, and T.L. Veum. 2000. Growth promotion effects and plasma changes from feeding high dietary concentrations of zinc and copper to weanling pigs (regional study). Journal of Animal Science 78, 1010-1016.

Hinton, M., and A.H. Linton. 1988. Control of Salmonella infections in broiler chickens by the acid treatment of their feed. The Veterinary Record 123, 416-421.

Hirn, J., E. Nurmi, T. Johansson, and L. Nuotio. 1992. Long-term experience with competitive exclusion and salmonellas in Finland. International Journal of Food Microbiology 15, 281-285.

Houdijk J.G.M. 1998. Effects of non-digestible oligosaccharides in young pig diets. PhD Thesis. Wageningen Agricultural University, The Netherlands

Hume, M.E., D.E. Corrier, S. Ambrus, A. Hinton, Jr., and J.R. DeLoach. 1993a. Effectiveness of dietary propionic acid in controlling Salmonella typhimurium colonization in broiler chicks. Avian Diseases 37, 1051-1056.

Hume, M.E., D.E. Corrier, G.W. Ivie, and J.R. Deloach. 1993b. Metabolism of [14C]propionic acid in broiler chicks. Poultry Science 72, 786-793.

Hume, M.E., J.A. Byrd, L.H. Stanker, and R.L. Ziprin. 1998. Reduction of caecal Listeria monocytogenes in Leghorn chicks following treatment with a competitive exclusion culture (PREEMPT). Letters in Applied Microbiology 26, 432-436.

Humphrey, T.J., and D.G. Lanning. 1988. The vertical transmission of salmonellas and formic acid treatment of chicken feed: A possible strategy for control. Epidemiology and Infection 100, 43-49.

Impey, C.S., G.C. Mead, and S.M. George. 1982. Competitive exclusion of salmonellas from the chick caecum using a defined mixture of bacterial isolates from the caecal microflora of an adult bird. Journal of Hygiene (Cambridge) 89, 479-490.

Isolauri, E., H. Majamaa, T. Arvola, I. Rantala, E. Virtanen, and H. Arvilommi. 1993. Lactobacillus casei strain GG reverses increased intestinal permeability induced by cow milk in suckling rats. Gastroenterology 105, 1643-1650.

Izat, A.L., N.M. Tidwell, R.A. Thomas, M.A. Reiber, M.H. Adams, M. Colberg, and P.W. Waldroup. 1990. Effects of a buffered propionic acid in diets on the performance of broiler chickens and on microflora of the intestine and carcass. Poultry Science 69, 818-826.

Jansen, G.J., A.C. Wildeboer-Veloo, R.H. Tonk, A.H. Franks, and G.W. Welling. 1999. Development and validation of an automated, microscopy-based method for enumeration of groups of intestinal bacteria. Journal of Microbiological Methods 37, 215-221.

Jensen-Waern, M., L. Melin, R. Lindberg, A. Johannisson, L. Petersson, and P. Wallgren. 1998. Dietary zinc oxide in weaned pigs—effects on performance, tissue concentrations, morphology, neutrophil functions and faecal microflora. Research in Veterinary Science 64, 225-231.

Kageyama, A., M. Sakamoto, and Y. Benno. 2000. Rapid identification and quantification of Collinsella aerofaciens using PCR. FEMS Microbiology Letters 183, 43-47.

Katouli, M., L. Melin, M. Jensen-Waern, P. Wallgren, and R. Mollby. 1999. The effect of zinc oxide supplementation on the stability of the intestinal flora with special reference to composition of coliforms in weaned pigs. Journal of Applied Microbiology 87, 564-573.

Kenworthy, R., and W.E. Crabb. 1963. The intestinal flora of young pigs with reference to early weaning and Escherischia coli scours. Journal of Comparative Pathology 73, 215-228.

Kimura, K., A.L. McCartney, M.A. McConnell, and G.W. Tannock. 1997. Analysis of faecal populations of bifidobacteria and lactobacilli and investigation of the immunological responses of their human hosts to the predominant strains. Applied & Environmental Microbiology 63, 3394-3398.

Kluger, M.J., C.A. Conn, B. Franklin, R. Freter, and G.D. Abrams. 1990. Effect of gastrointestinal flora on body temperature of rats and mice. American Journal of Physiology 258, R552-557.

Koopman, J.P., H.M. Kennis, J.W. Mullink, R.A. Prins, A.M. Stadhouders, H. De Boer, and M.P. Hectors. 1984. 'Normalization' of germfree mice with anaerobically cultured caecal flora of 'normal' mice. Laboratory Animals 18, 188-194.

Langendijk, P.S.,F. Schut, G.J. Jansen, G.C. Raangs, G.R. Kamphuis, M.H. Wilkinson, and G.W. Welling. 1995. Quantitative fluorescence in situ hybridization of Bifidobacterium spp. with genus-specific 16S rRNA-targeted probes and its application in faecal samples. Applied & Environmental Microbiology 61, 3069-3075.

Licht, T.R., K.A. Krogfelt, P.S. Cohen, L.K. Poulsen, J. Urbance, and S. Molin. 1996. Role of lipopolysaccharide in colonization of the mouse intestine by Salmonella typhimurium studied by in situ hybridization. Infection & Immunity 64, 3811-3817.

Lin, C., L. Raskin, and D.A. Stahl. 1997. Microbial community structure in gastrointestinal tracts of domestic animals: comparative analyses using rRNA-targeted oligonucleotide probes. FEMS Microbiology and Ecology 22, 281-294.

Lowden, S., and T. Heath. 1995. Segmented filamentous bacteria associated with lymphoid tissues in the ileum of horses. Research in Veterinary Science 59, 272-274.

Ludwig, W., and K.-H. Schleifer. 2000. How quantitative is quantitative PCR with respect to cell counts? Systematic and Applied Microbiology 23, 556-562.

Mackie, R., A. Sghir, and H.R. Gaskins. 1999. Developmental microbial ecology of the neonatal gastrointestinal tract. American Journal of Clinical Nutrition 69, 1035S-1045S.

Mallett, A.K., and I.R. Rowland. 1988. Factors affecting the gut microflora. In I. R. Rowland (ed.), Role of the Gut Flora in Toxicity and Cancer. Academic Press, London. pp. 347-382.

Mantere-Alhonen, S. 1995. Propionibacteria used as probiotics - A review. Le Lait 75, 447-452.

Mathers, J.C., and E.F. Annison. 1993. Stoichiometry of polysaccharide fermentation in the large intestine. In: S. Samman and G. Annison (ed.), *Dietary Fibre and Beyond-Australian Perspectives*, vol. 1. Nutrition Society of Australia Occasional Publications. pp. 123-135.

Mathew, A.G., A.L. Sutton, A.B. Scheidt, J.A. Patterson, D.T. Kelly, and K.A. Meyerholtz. 1993. Effect of galactan on selected microbial populations and pH and volatile fatty acids in the ileum of the weanling pig. Journal of Animal Science 71, 1503-1509.

McHan, F., and E.B. Shotts. 1992. Effect of feeding selected short-chain fatty acids on the *in vivo* attachment of *Salmonella typhimurium* in chick ceca. Avian Diseases 36, 139-142.

Mead, G.C., and B.W. Adams. 1975. Some observations on the caecal microflora of the chick during the first two weeks of life. British Poultry Science 16, 169-176.

Mead, G.C., and P.A. Barrow. 1990. Salmonella control in poultry by 'competitive exclusion' or immunization. Letters in Applied Microbiology 10, 221-227.

Mead, G.C., M.J. Scott, T.J. Humphrey, and K. McAlpine. 1996. Observations on the control of Campylobacter jejuni infection of poultry by competitive exclusion. Avian Pathology 25, 69-79.

Metchnikoff, E. 1907. The Prolongation of Life. Optimistic Studies. William Heinemann, London.

Metchnikoff, E. 1908. The Nature of Man. Studies in Optimistic Philosophy. William Heinemann, London.

Miles, R.D., S.F. O'Keefe, P.R. Henry, C.B. Ammerman, and X. G. Luo. 1998. The effect of dietary supplementation with copper sulfate or tribasic copper chloride on broiler performance, relative copper bioavailability, and dietary prooxidant activity. Poultry Science 77, 416-425.

Millar, M.R., C. Bacon, S.L. Smith, V. Walker, and M.A. Hall. 1993. Enteral feeding of premature infants with Lactobacillus GG. Archives of Diseases in Children 69, 2595-2600.

Moore, W.E., and L.V. Holdeman. 1974. Human faecal flora: the normal flora of 20 Japanese-Hawaiians. Applied Microbiology 27, 961-979.

Mulder, R.W.A.W., and N.M. Bolder. 1991a. Experience with competitive exclusion in the Netherlands, In: L.C. Blankenship (ed.), Colonization control of human bacterial enteropathogens in poultry. Academic Press, San Diego. pp. 77-89.

Mulder, R.W.A.W., and N.M. Bolder. 1991b. Reduction of Campylobacter infection of broilers by competitive exclusion treatment of day-old broiler chicks — A field study. In: L.C. Blankenship (ed.), Colonization control of human bacterial enteropathogens in poultry. Academic Press, San Diego. pp. 359-363.

Mulder, R.W.A.W., R. Havenaar, and J.H.J. Huis in 't Veld. 1997. Intervention strategies: the use of probiotics and competitive exclusion microfloras against contamination with pathogens in poultry and pigs. In: R. Fuller (ed.), Probiotics 2: Application and practical aspects. Chapman & Hall, New York. pp. 187-207.

Muyzer, G., and K. Smalla. 1998. Application of denaturing gradient gel electrophoresis (DGGE) and temperature gradient gel electrophoresis (TGGE) in microbial ecology. Antonie Van Leeuwenhoek 73, 127-141.

Nelson, G.M., and S.E. George. 1995. Comparison of media for selection and enumeration of mouse faecal flora populations. Journal of Microbiological Methods 22:293-300.

Nemcova, R., A. Bomba, S. Gancarcikova, R. Herich, and P. Guba. 1999. Study of the effect of Lactobacillus paracasei and fructooligosaccharides on the faecal microflora in weanling piglets. Berliner und Münchener Tierarztlichen Wochenschrift 112(6-7):225-228.

Nisbet, D.J., D.E. Corrier, C.M. Scanlan, A.G. Hollister, R.C. Beier, and J.R. DeLoach. 1993. Effect of a defined continuous-flow derived bacterial culture and dietary lactose on *Salmonella typhimurium* colonization in broiler chickens. Avian Diseases 37, 1017-1025.

Nisbet, D.J., D.E. Corrier, S.C. Ricke, M.E. Hume, I. Byrd, J.A., and J.R. DeLoach. 1996. Caecal propionic acid as a biological indicator of the early establishment of a microbial ecosystem inhibitory to Salmonella in chicks. Anaerobe 2, 345-350.

Nuotio, L., C. Schneitz, U. Halonen, and E. Nurmi. 1992. Use of competitive exclusion to protect newly-hatched chicks against intestinal colonisation and invasion by *Salmonella enteritidis* PT4. British Poultry Science 33, 775-779.

Nurmi, E., and M. Rantale. 1973. New aspects of Salmonella infection in broiler production. Nature 241, 210-211.

Ofek, I., D. Mirelman, and N. Sharon. 1977. Adherence of Escherichia coli to human mucosal cells mediated by mannose receptors. Nature 265, 623-5.

Opitz, A.M., M. El-Begearmi, P. Flegg, and D. Beane. 1993. Effectiveness of five feed additives in chicks infected with *Salmonella enteritidis* phage type 13A. Journal of Applied Poultry Research 2, 147-153.

Ouwehand, A.C., and S.J. Salminen. 1998. The health effects of cultured milk products with viable and non-viable bacteria. International Dairy Journal 8, 749-758.

Palmu, L., and I. Camelin. 1997. The use of competitive exclusion in broilers to reduce the level of Salmonella contamination on the farm and at the processing plant. Poultry Science 76, 1501-1505.

Pascual, M., M. Hugas, J.I. Badiola, J.M. Monfort, and M. Garriga. 1999. Lactobacillus salivarius CTC2197 prevents Salmonella enteritidis colonization in chickens. Applied & Environmental Microbiology 65, 4981-4986.

Pollmann, D.S., E.R. Danielson, and E.R. Peo, jr. 1980. Effects of microbial feed additives on performance of starter and growth-finishing pigs. Journal of Animal Science 51, 577.

Pryde, S.E., A.J. Richardson, C.S. Stewart, and H.J. Flint. 1999. Molecular analysis of the microbial diversity present in the colonic wall, colonic lumen, and caecal lumen of a pig. Applied and Environmental Microbiology 65: 5372-5377.

Pusztai A., G. Grant, R.J. Spencer, T.J. Duguid, D.S. Brown, S.W.B. Ewen, W.J. Peumans, E.J.M. Van Damme, and S. Bardocz. 1993. Kidney bean lectin-induced Escherichia coli overgrowth in the small intestine is blocked by GNA, a mannose-specific lectin. Journal of Applied Bacteriology 75: 360-368.

Rantale, M., and E. Nurmi. 1973. Prevention of the growth of *Salmonella infantis* in chicks by the flora of the alimentary tract of chickens. British Poultry Science 14, 627-630.

Rowland, I.R. 1992. Metabolic interactions in the gut. Probiotics- The Scientific Basis. Chapman & Hall, London. pp. 29-53

Salvat, G., F. Lalande, F. Humbert, and C. Lahellec. 1992. Use of a competitive exclusion product (Broilact) to prevent Salmonella colonization of newly hatched chicks. International Journal of Food Microbiology 15, 307-311.

Sanford, S.E. 1991. Light and electron microscopic observations of a segmented filamentous bacterium attached to the mucosa of the terminal ileum of pigs. Journal of Veterinary Diagnostics and Investigations 3, 328-333.

Satokari, R.M., E.E. Vaughan, A.D. Akkermans, M. Saarela, and W.M. de Vos. 2001. Bifidobacterial diversity in human feces detected by genus-specific pcr and denaturing gradient gel electrophoresis. Applied & Environmental Microbiology 67, 504-513.

Savage, D.C. 1977. Microbial ecology of the gastrointestinal tract. Annual Reviews in Microbiology 31, 107-133.

Schoeni, J.L., and A.C. L. Wong. 1994. Inhibition of Campylobacter jejuni colonization in chicks by defined competitive exclusion bacteria. Applied & Environmental Microbiology 60, 1191-1197.

Sepp, E., M. Mikelsaar, and S. Salminen. 1993. Effect of administration of Lactobacillus casei strain GG on the gastrointestinal microbionta of newborns. Microbiology and Ecology in Health and Disease 6, 309-314.

Sghir, A., D. Antonopoulos, and R.I. Mackie. 1998. Design and evaluation of a Lactobacillus group-specific ribosomal RNA- targeted hybridization probe and its application to the study of intestinal microecology in pigs. Systematic and Applied Microbiology 21, 291-296.

Simmering, R., B. Kleessen, and M. Blaut. 1999. Quantification of the flavonoid-degrading bacterium Eubacterium ramulus in human faecal samples with a species-specific oligonucleotide hybridization probe. Applied & Environmental Microbiology 65, 3705-3709.

Simpson, J.M., V.J. McCracken, B.A. White, H.R. Gaskins, and R.I. Mackie. 1999. Application of denaturant gradient gel electrophoresis for the analysis of the porcine gastrointestinal microbiota. Journal of Microbiological Methods 36, 167-179.

Smith, T.M. 1997. Segmented filamentous bacteria in the bovine small intestine. Journal of Comparative Pathology 117, 185-190.

Snel, J., C.C. Hermsen, H.J. Smits, N.A. Bos, W.M. Eling, J.J. Cebra, and P.J. Heidt. 1998. Interactions between gut-associated lymphoid tissue and colonization levels of indigenous, segmented, filamentous bacteria in the small intestine of mice. Canadian Journal of Microbiology 44, 1177-1182.

Snel, J., J. Hoolwerf, M. Wissink, I. Bovee-Oudenhoven, R. Van der Meer, and A. Herrewegh. 2000. Use of quantitative PCR to demonstrate effects of prebiotics on intestinal lactobacilli and salmonella. "Functional food challenges for the new millenium". 5th Karlsruhe Nutrition Congress held in Karlsruhe, October 22-24. p. 21

Soerjadi, A.S., S.M. Stehman, G.H. Snoeyenbos, O.M. Weinack, and C.F. Smyser. 1981. The influence of Lactobacilli on the competitive exclusion of parathypoid Salmonellae in chickens. Avian Diseases 25, 1027-1033.

Soerjardi-Liem, A.S., G.H. Snoeyenbos, and O.M. Weinack. 1984. Comparative studies on competitive exclusion of three isolates of Campylobacter fetus subsp. jejuni in chickens by native gut microflora. Avian Diseases 28, 139-146.

Stavric, S., T.M. Gleeson, B. Blanchfield, and H. Pivnick. 1985. Competitive exclusion of Salmonella from newly hatched chicks by mixtures of pure bacterial cultures isolated from faecal and caecal contents of adult birds. Journal of Food Protection 48, 778-782.

Stavric, S., T.M. Gleeson, and B. Blanchfield. 1991. Effect of avian intestinal microflora possessing adhering and hydrophobic properties on competitive exclusion of Salmonella typhimurium from chicks. Journal of Applied Bacteriology 70, 414-421.

Steer, T., H. Carpenter, K. Tuohy, and G.R. Gibson. 2000. Perspectives on the role of the human gut microbiota and its modulation by pro- and pre-biotics. Nutrition Research Reviews 13, 229-254.

Stern, N.J. 1994. Mucosal competitive exclusion to diminish colonization of chickens by Campylobacter jejuni. Poultry Science 73, 402-407.

Stewart, C.S., K. Hillman, F. Maxwell, D. Kelly, and T.P. King. 1993. Recent advances in probiosis in pigs: observations on the microbiology of the pig gut. In: P.C. Garnsworthy and D.J.A. Cole (ed.), Recent Advances in Animal Nutrition. Nottingham University Press. pp. 197-220

Tannock, G.W., K. Munro, H.J. Harmsen, G.W. Welling, J. Smart, and P.K. Gopal. 2000. Analysis of the faecal microflora of human subjects consuming a probiotic product containing Lactobacillus rhamnosus DR20. Applied & Environmental Microbiology 66, 2578-2588.

Thompson, J.L., and M. Hinton. 1997. Antibacterial activity of formic and propionic acids in the diet of hens on Salmonellas in the crop. British Poultry Science 38, 59-65.

Tortuero, F., J. Rioperez, E. Fernandez, and M.L. Rodriguez. 1995. Response of piglets to oral administration of lactic acid bacteria. Journal of Food. Protection 58, 1369-1374.

Umesaki, Y. 1989. Intestinal glycolipids and their possible role in microbial colonization of mice. Bifidobacteria Microflora 8, 13-22.

Umesaki, Y., H. Setoyama, S. Matsumoto, and Y. Okada. 1993. Expansion of alpha beta T-cell receptor-bearing intestinal intraepithelial lymphocytes after microbial colonization in germ-free mice and its independence from thymus. Immunology 79, 32-37.

Umesaki, Y., Y. Okada, A. Imaoka, H. Setoyama, and S. Matsumoto. 1997. Interactions between epithelial cells and bacteria, normal and pathogenic. Science 276, 964-965.

Van der Waaij, D., J.M. Berghuis-de Vries, and J.E. Lekkerkerk-Van der Wees. 1971. Colonization resistance of the digestive tract in conventional and antibiotic-treated mice. Journal of Hygiene (Lond) 69, 405-411.

Van der Wielen, P.W.J.J., S. Biesterveld, S. Notermans, H. Hofstra, B.A.P. Urlings, and F. van Knapen. 2000. Role of Volatile Fatty Acids in Development of the Caecal Microflora in Broiler Chickens during Growth. Applied & Environmental Microbiology 66, 2536-2540.

Van der Wielen, P.W.J.J., S. Biesterveld, L.J.A. Lipman, and F. Van Knapen. 2001. Inhibition of a glucose limited sequencing fed-batch culture of Salmonella enterica serovar Enteritidis by volatile fatty acids representative for the ceca of broilers. Applied & Environmental Micriobiology 67, 1979-1982.

Ward, D.M., M.M. Bateson, R. Weller, and A.L. Ruff-Roberts. 1992. Ribosomal RNA analysis of microorganisms as they occur in nature, vol. 12. Plenum Press, New York. pp. 219-286

Weinack, O.M., G.H. Snoeyenbos, and A.S. Soerjadi-Liem. 1985. Further studies on competitive exclusion of Salmonella typhimurium by lactobacilli in chickens. Avian Diseases 29, 1273-1276.

Wierup, M.,H. Wahlstrom, and B. Engstrom. 1992. Experience of a 10-year use of competitive exclusion treatment as part of the Salmonella control programme in Sweden. International Journal of Food Microbiology 15, 287-291.

Williams, B.A., M. Bosch, J. Houdijk, and Y. Van de Camp. 1997a. Differences in potential fermentative capablilities of four sections of porcine digestive tract., Proc 48th EAAP meeting held in Vienna August 25-29. Abst. 195.

Williams, B.A., L.J.M. Van Osch, and R.P. Kwakkel. 1997b. Fermentation characteristics of the caecal contents of broiler chickens fed fine- and coarse particle diets. WPSA Spring Meeting (UK Branch) Scarborough, 26- 27 March. p. 49

Williams, B.A., S. Tamminga, and M.W.A. Verstegen. 2000a. Fermentation kinetics to assess microbial activity of gastro-intestinal microflora. In: Proceedings of the symposium "Gas Production: Fermentation kinetics for feed evaluation and to assess microbial activity" held in Wageningen, Netherlands August 18-19. pp. 97-100

Williams, B.A., W.-Y. Zhu, A. Akkermans, and S. Tamminga. 2000b. An *in vitro* test for prebiotics, , "Challanges for microbial digestive ecology" 2nd joint INRA-RRI Gastrointestinal Tract Microbiology Symposium held in Clermont-Ferrand, May 25-26. Abst. 225

Williams, B.A., M.W.A. Verstegen, and S. Tamminga. 2001. Fermentation in the monogastric large intestine: its relation to animal health. Nutrition Research Reviews, in press.

Wilson, K.H., and R.B. Blitchington. 1996. Human colonic biota studied by ribosomal DNA sequence analysis. Applied & Environmental Microbiology 62, 2273-2278.

Yokoyama, M.T., C. Tabori, E.R. Miller, and M.G. Hogberg. 1982. The effects of antibiotics in the weanling pig diet on growth and the excretion of volatile phenolic and aromatic bacterial metabolites. American Journal of Clinical Nutrition 35, 1417-1424.

Zhao, T., M.P. Doyle, B.G. Harmon, C.A. Brown, P.O. Mueller, and A.H. Parks. 1998. Reduction of carriage of enterohemorrhagic Escherichia coli O157:H7 in cattle by inoculation with probiotic bacteria. Journal of Clinical Microbiology 36, 641-647.

Ziprin, R.L., D.E. Corrier, A. Hinton, jr., R.C. Beier, G.E. Spates, J.R. DeLoach, and M.H. Elissalde. 1990. Intracloacal Salmonella typhimurium infection of broiler chickens: Reduction of colonization with anaerobic organisms and dietary lactose. Avian Diseases 34, 749-753.

Zoetendal, E.G., A.D.L. Akkermans, and W.M. De Vos. 1998. Temperature gradient gel electrophoresis analysis of 16S rRNA from human faecal samples reveals stable and host-specific communities of active bacteria. Applied & Environmental Microbiology 64, 3854-3859.

Zulkifli, I., N. Abdullah, N. Mohd.Azrin, and Y.W. Ho. 2000. Growth performance and immune response of two commercial broiler strains fed diets containing Lactobacillus cultures and oxytetracycline under heat stress conditions. British Poultry Science 41, 593-597.

3. Structural and functional aspects of a healthy gastrointestinal tract

J.E. van Dijk[1], J. Huisman[2], J.F.J.G. Koninkx[1]
[1] *Department of Pathology, Faculty of Veterinary Medicine, Utrecht University, Yalelaan 1, P.O. Box 80158, 3508 TD Utrecht, The Netherlands*
[2] *ID TNO Animal Nutrition, P.O. Box 65, 8200 AB Lelystad, The Netherlands*

Summary

The macroscopic and microscopic morphology in relation to function of the gastrointestinal mucosal epithelium with its mucus layer and some regulatory mechanisms are discussed. Attention is paid to the role of age of the organism and characteristics of the feed (short chain fatty acids, lectins) for length of the intestine, height of villi and depth of crypts, regulation of proliferation and functional maturation of enterocytes and composition of mucins in goblet cells. Some deleterious as well as advantageous effects of feed components, feed additives and microflora on structure and function of the mucosal epithelium are mentioned. The influence of dietary components on repair, defence and resistance of the intestinal mucosa is discussed. Possibilities to draw conclusions on intestinal health based on the *in vivo* and *in vitro* structure of intestinal cells are presented.
Based on the regulatory mechanisms in the intestine the use of feed additives and pro- and prebiotics to improve resistance and to stabilise intestinal health is commented.

3.1. Introduction

The gastrointestinal tract has different possibilities to adapt or to react morphologically to changing conditions such as for instance birth (Puchal et al., 1992; Cranwell, 1995, Sangild, 2000), weaning (Van Beers-Schreurs et al., 1998), altered diet (Huisman et al., 1990; Van der Klis et al., 1993) or altered composition of the intestinal microflora (Koninkx et al., 1988; Kelly et al., 2001). The intestine can change its surface by growing in length, and/or by increasing or decreasing the height of its villi. Shortening and fusion of villi will result in loss of surface for digestion and absorption of food. Moreover, the morphology of each individual epithelial intestinal cell (enterocyte, crypt cell, goblet cell, endocrine cell) is not rigid but is function related. In the healthy gut these differences have spatial and temporal patterns; they are related to the place along the duodenal-jejunal-ileal axis and the crypt-villus axis and to the age of the organism (Buddington, 1997; Pluske, 2001). So, nature has defined a variety of functional and morphological solutions to provide the intestinal mucosa with optimal properties, given the circumstances. The attention in this paper will mainly be focused on the mucosa of the small intestine of mammals, but relevant functional aspects of the large intestine will be included and many aspects are also valid for other animals.

The enormous increase of surface of the small intestinal mucosa is possible due to the presence of mucosal projections as ridges, folds, (zigzag) lamellae or villi. In farm mammals mainly finger-like villi projecting into the intestinal lumen are found in the small intestine (Figure 1) and in chickens also in caeca, colon and rectum. In conventional animals fused villi and in poultry even lamellae, are often seen. Glands or crypts are present between the projections. Epithelial cells, the enterocytes, cover the villi. The microvilli of these cells accomplish an additional significant increase of

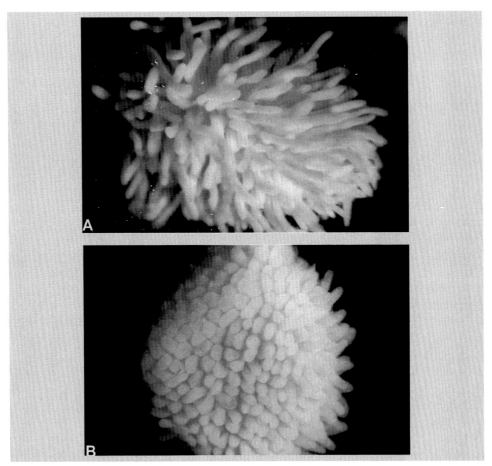

Figure 1. Biopsies showing the luminal surface of bovine jejunal intestine of SPF-animals.
Finger-like villi are present in control bovine jejunal biopsies (A) and shortened, sometimes fused villi after feeding a Glycine max agglutinin (SBA) containing diet (B).

the mucosal surface. Diminishment of number or quality of (micro) villi is a frequent finding and can be caused by food substances and many microorganisms. The epithelial cells on the villi are continuously replaced by proliferation in the crypts, migration of cells from the crypts up to the villi and eventually after 3-6 days apoptosis or exfoliation (shedding) at the villus tips.

During migration most of the immature crypt cells differentiate and become mature enterocytes on the villi. Other cells become endocrine or mucin producing cells (Mouwen et al., 1983). This layer of epithelial cells, together with the mucus layer on top of it and the basal lamina beneath, provides digestion, selective permeability and the major part of its resistance. The mucus layer and the epithelial cell layer constitute the first line of defence; it is immediately active and almost non-specific, although the presence of secretory immuno-globulins (Goddeeris et al., Chapter 4 of this publication) in the mucus also warrants a specific defence.

3.2. Mucus layer

The mucus layer is a viscous secretion, which, in the intestine, is mainly synthesised by goblet cells. It consists of a continuous layer, about 400 µm in thickness that covers the villi. After fixation and staining dehydration, denaturation and severe and variable shrinkage have occurred. The viscosity results from non-covalent interactions between large and highly hydrated glycoconjugates. These glycoconjugates or mucins have a (small) peptide core with many and long, often branched, side-chains of sugars. At the end of the synthesis-pathway the terminal sugars of the mucins may become sulphated or sialylated, resulting in acidic mucins. Acidic mucins are more resistant to microbiological degradation than newly formed, neutral mucins. Especially the long and branched chains can become sulphated, whereas shorter and more linear chains can become sialylated (Mantle et al., 1989).

Changes in the quantitative and qualitative characteristics of the mucus layer can be caused by changes in synthesis and/or degradation. This can be demonstrated in a model in which rats are experimentally infected with *Nippostrongylus brasiliensis* (Koninkx et al., 1988a). There are striking changes in the synthesis of mucins in the rat small intestine after infection with this nematode parasite. With respect to the synthesis of mucins, not only an increase in the number of goblet cells is found after infection, but the composition of mucins in the goblet cells, as determined by histochemical criteria, is also subject to changes (Table 1). The AB-PAS stain enables to distinguish between neutral and acid mucins and the HID-AB stain between sulpho- and sialomucins.

It is known that synthesis of mucins and staining characteristics of mucins in the goblet cells correlate with (lack of) differentiation or (im)maturity of the goblet cells in disease, particularly in malignancy (Ehsanullah et al., 1982; Reid et al., 1984; Turani et al.; 1986). Immature goblet cells of intestinal neoplasms and foetal intestinal cells produce neutral and still incomplete mucins. Also after infection with nematodes at 6 and 10 days under conditions of increased proliferation of crypt cells (Figure 2), the synthesised mucins express the immaturity of both crypt and villus goblet cells

Table 1. Staining Characteristics of Goblet Cell Mucins of the Jejunal Villi and Crypts at Different Times after Subcutaneous Inoculation with 4000 Infective Larvae of *Nippostrongylus brasiliensis*

Days after inoculation	Number of rats	Number of goblet cells containing acid mucins, neutral mucins, or a mixture of acid and neutral mucins			Number of goblet cells containing sialomucins, sulfomucins, or a mixture of sialo- and sulfomucins		
		Acid	Acid/neutral	Neutral	Sialo	Sialo/sulfo	Sulfo
Crypt							
Control	12	9.8 ± 1.2	2.9 ± 0.6	1.4 ± 0.4	7.2 ± 0.8	4.5 ± 0.8	2.3 ± 0.7
6	12	12.2 ± 3.1[a]	6.7 ± 1.0[a]	4.5 ± 0.9[a]	5.8 ± 1.5[a]	12.3 ± 2.3[a]	5.2 ± 1.6[a]
10	12	14.8 ± 1.3[ab]	16.7 ± 1.1[ab]	7.5 ± 0.7[ab]	6.8 ± 1.0**	16.0 ± 1.2[ab]	16.2 ± 1.4[ab]
15	12	29.6 ± 2.7[abc]	5.0 ± 0.9[abc]	0.3 ± 0.2[abc]	0.3 ± 0.1[abc]	2.6 ± 0.6[abc]	32.1 ± 3.3[abc]
20	12	16.7 ± 1.1[abcd]	3.9 ± 0.6[abcd]	0.8 ± 0.3[abcd]	3.0 ± 0.9[abcd]	12.3 ± 1.3[a*cd]	6.0 ± 1.3[a*cd]
Villus							
Control	12	18.0 ± 1.4	6.6 ± 0.5	1.9 ± 0.2	14.9 ± 1.1	8.8 ± 0.7	2.9 ± 0.2
6	12	26.2 ± 2.2[a]	6.5 ± 0.5*	3.6 ± 0.3[a]	10.2 ± 0.8[a]	22.1 ± 1.8[a]	4.0 ± 0.3[a]
10	12	19.0 ± 1.3*[b]	16.2 ± 1.1[ab]	5.3 ± 0.4[ab]	9.3 ± 0.6[ab]	20.2 ± 1.3[ab]	10.9 ± 0.7[ab]
15	12	36.3 ± 2.3[abc]	4.5 ± 0.3[abc]	0.5 ± 0.1[abc]	0.4 ± 0.1[abc]	3.3 ± 0.2[abc]	37.6 ± 2.4[abc]
20	12	20.5 ± 2.2[ab*d]	5.6 ± 0.6[abcd]	0.5 ± 0.1[abc*]	2.4 ± 0.3[abcd]	15.4 ± 1.7[abcd]	8.8 ± 1.0[abcd]

Note. The number of differently stained goblet cells determined in 10 well-oriented villi and crypts per rat, is indicated. The mean ± SD is presented

[a] a significant difference with control rats ($P < 0.05$)

[b] a significant difference with rats 6 days after infection ($P < 0.05$)

[c] a significant difference with rats 10 days after infection ($P < 0.05$)

[d] a significant difference with rats 20 days after infection ($P < 0.05$)

An asterisk * at the position [abcd] indicates that with respect to that item no significant difference exists

(After Koninkx et al., 1988)

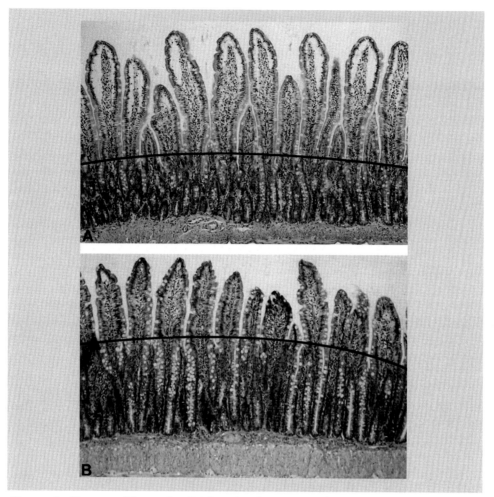

Figure 2. Hematoxilin-eosin (HE)-stained rat jejunal sections to demonstrate changes in villus height, crypt depth and number of goblet cells.
Control rats (A) and Nippostrongylus brasiliensis infected rats (10 days post-infection) (B). The line approximately indicates the villus-crypt border (Magnification x425).

(Koninkx et al., 1988a). The observed increase at 15 days after infection in the number of acid mucin-containing goblet cells appears to be due to an increase in the number of sulphomucin-containing goblet cells. As is the case in colonic carcinogenesis (Filipe et al., 1979; Forstner et al., 1982) normal regulatory mechanisms of mucin synthesis are probably influenced in rats after infection with Nippostrongylus brasiliensis. As a result an at least temporary adaptation of mucin synthesis takes place. There is a striking correlation between worm expulsion and hyperplasia of goblet cells (Ferguson et al., 1975). The data presented in table 1 confirm this finding and, in addition, clearly show that the nature of the mucins in the goblet cells changes from neutral to acid (sulphated) between 10 and 15 days after infection. These quantitative and qualitative changes in synthesis of mucins, which coincide with expulsion of worms, most probably interfere with the physicochemical properties of the mucus layer on the mucosal surface. The thus modified mucus (Forstner et al., 1982) might render increased protection against and facilitates expulsion of the nematode worms.

In a study of van Leeuwen et al. (2001) the mucin type in goblet cells of the crypts was evaluated in piglets fed a control diet (n=5) without antibiotics, and a group fed a diet supplemented with 40 ppm virginiamycin (n=5), respectively. Three weeks after weaning the piglets were challenged with E. coli K88. One week post challenge samples of the small intestinal mucosa were taken and animal growth over this period was measured. The percentages of goblet cells with sulphomucins (positive HID-stain) of both groups were similar. However, correlation analysis showed a negative correlation between daily weight gain and the percentage of HID$^+$ crypt goblet cells of the proximal part of the small intestine (P<0.05; R^2= 0.7) (Figure 3). This result indicated that the sulphated mucin type enhances the protective function of the mucus when (sub) clinical infections occur. Also litter effects (P<0.1) were observed regarding numbers of crypt goblet cells and mucin type in the crypt goblet cells. This may imply that variation in the small intestinal architecture between piglets is related with the genetic background of the piglets (and, possibly, may have implications for bacterial attachment to glycoproteins of the brush border membrane). In the same piglets a significant correlation was found between daily weight gain and villus length (Figure 4).

The mucus layer shows two distinct physical forms; first, a thin, very viscous and water insoluble layer of gel which firmly adheres to the epithelial surface and, second, a soluble component on top of it. Especially in this soluble layer ingested material at various stages of digestion is present, but also enzymes, adhering micro-organisms and immunoglobulins (IgA). Together, the two layers are often referred to as unstirred

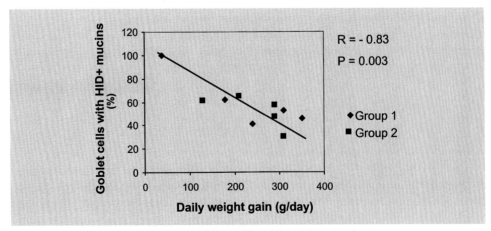

Figure 3. Daily weight gain vs goblet cells with HID+ mucins.
Group 1 is fed a control diet and group 2 a diet containing 40 ppm virginiamycin.

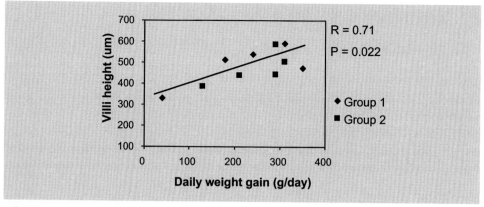

Figure 4. Daily weight gain vs villus height.
Group 1 is fed a control diet and group 2 a diet containing 40 ppm virginiamycin.

water layer (UWL). The mucus layer is susceptible to proteolytic digestion by digestive and microbial enzymes; this explains the conversion of the deeper gel layer to viscous fluid on top. The balance between secretion and degradation determines the thickness of the mucus layer. In addition to the baseline secretion parasympathetic and chemical stimulation or mediators of inflammatory reactions, such as products of T lymphocytes may stimulate the mucin secretion. Addition of highly viscous carboxymethylcellulose, a non-digestible polysaccharide, to the diet of growing chickens resulted in beneficial morphological effects on the small intestinal mucosa (long villi, low mitotic activity) with high numbers of goblet cells indicating a higher production of mucus. However, the lipid, starch and nitrogen digestibility was depressed (Smits et al., 1996[a,b]). A longer distance for diffusion by an increased thickness of the mucus layer may be one of the reasons for this phenomenon. Degradation of mucus depends on several factors, including intestinal flora, mechanical injury, digestive enzymes, gastric acid and bile. So, a dynamic equilibrium exists between secretion and degradation as well as between the tough gel layer and the water-soluble upper layer (Lamont, 1992; Mouwen et al., 1983).

Summarising, the mucus layer enables passage of intestinal contents by lubrication of the intestinal surface and it constitutes a first barrier for chemical, microbiological or physical injury of the underlying enterocytes. Damage or removal of the mucus layer gives access to the apical membrane of the enterocytes and excessive binding of unwanted ligands to receptors in that membrane can result. Changes in quantity or quality of mucus can be expected in all conditions affecting the proliferation or differentiation of intestinal epithelial cells, from crypt to villus. These conditions may be the normal resident microflora (Kelly et al., 2001), pathogens or non-infectious agents, such as methotrexate (Koninkx et al., 1988b) or a diet supplemented with enzymes (Fernandez et al., 2000). Increase of thickness of the mucus layer may protect the enterocyte but the longer distance for diffusion before terminal digestion and absorption takes place may hamper an optimal utilisation of the food.

3.3. Enterocytes

3.3.1. Developments during early life

Size and number of enterocytes are strongly variable. Immediately after birth of a mammal the intestine strongly increases in weight, mainly of the mucosa. This rapid weight gain is not only caused by hypertrophy of the enterocytes due to non-selective endocytosis of colostral immunoglobulins and other macromolecules (hormones, growth factors), but also as a result of increased protein synthesis and crypt cell hyperplasia (Xu et al., 1992). At this time secretion of pancreatic enzymes is low and proteinase inhibitors are present in the colostrum (Weström, 1997). In piglets and calves intestinal closure occurs abruptly, 18-36 h after birth. After that time only absorption of molecules less than a few kilo-Dalton is possible. Uptake of larger macromolecules into enterocytes will proceed for some time, but these molecules remain in the fetal-type enterocytes for intracellular breakdown or storage until shedding. These fetal enterocytes are gradually replaced by adult-type enterocytes, a process that starts proximally and ends at last in the distal part of the small intestine at 3-4 weeks after birth. In rodents mainly a selective uptake of immunoglobulins takes place, after binding to Fc-receptors on enterocytes of the proximal intestine; intestinal closure is complete at weaning, about 3 weeks after birth. In man, macromolecular absorption is very limited (Weström, 1997). After weaning absorption of macromolecules is limited to abnormal conditions in the gut, with disruption of the tight junctions between adjacent enterocytes at the apical/basolateral boundary. Such leaky tight junctions induce the possibility of paracellular permeability for large molecules and may cause food allergy.

The enzymatic equipment of stomach and intestine changes considerably during the first 1-2 days after birth. Gastric acid production and pepsin activity are very low around birth, while the secretion of milk-clotting protease chymosin is at its maximum. At birth intestinal lactase shows a peak in activity and peptidases are already well developed. Lactase activity decreases during the first days, whereas maltase and aminopeptidases show a rapid increase. Driving forces for these developments are ingestion of amniotic fluid, glucocorticoid surge before and during parturition, and colostrum with hormones and growth factors (Sangild, 1997). At birth most enterocytes lining the villi are fully differentiated. In older animals only the upper one third of the villus is provided with fully differentiated enterocytes and therefore, rates of uptake of nutrients per mg of intestine or unit of intestinal length are higher at birth than at any other age (Smith, 1988). However, digestive or absorptive capacity of the small intestine should not be measured as activity per mg of intestine, but as activity of the entire (rapidly growing!) small intestine (Pusztai et al., 1996; Buddington, 1997).

Abrupt weaning induces lowered levels of food intake, shortening of villi and microvilli, deepening of crypts, and increased turnover of enterocytes (Van Beers-Schreurs et al., 1998; Buddington, 1997; Pluske, 2001). These changes are indicative for a diminished digestive and absorptive capacity. Maintenance of food intake can largely prevent these changes (Van Beers-Schreurs et al., 1998; Pluske, 2001). These data indicate that it is appropriate to prepare weaning diets for piglets with high content of highly digestible milk proteins to achieve high palatability resulting in good energy intake and good intestinal development. Other highly digestible proteins may also be of interest, for instance blood plasma proteins (Van Dijk, 2001, Van Dijk et al., 2001). However, there are also indications that he histological and morphological changes during weaning are independent of diet composition (McCracken et al., 1995).

3.3.2. Morphology and function of enterocytes

The enterocytes on the upper third of a villus are fully equipped for their digestive and absorptive function. They bear microvilli on their apical part bordering the gut lumen. Together the microvilli form the brush border. They have an outercoat called glycocalyx, which contains the sugar chains of glycoconjugates. Their protein cores are anchored in the plasma membrane of the enterocyte. Part of these glycoproteins represent digestive enzymes and absorptive transmembrane carrier proteins (Buddington, 1997). The poly-sugar chains of the glycocalyx may also serve as receptors for all kind of biologically active factors such as viruses, non-pathogenic and pathogenic bacteria, nutrients, lectins, toxins and biologically active hormones, growth factors and other peptides (Egberts et al., 1984; Sangild, 1997). The composition of the carbohydrate chains is extremely variable and offers many possibilities for adaptation. The binding characteristics of the glycoproteins depend on the type of exposed sugars and will change whenever these terminal sugars change. In this way the possibility of attachment of, for instance, growth factors, micro-organisms or lectins may increase or decrease (Egberts et al., 1984; Naughton, 2001). Similar glycoconjugates and carbohydrate binding proteins are found on microbial cells (Naughton, 2001).

The regulation of rate of proliferation and differentiation of enterocytes is complicated. Animal species, age, genetics and environmental influences, such as dietary components or intestinal resident microflora and pathogens are involved (Sangild, 1997; Pluske 2001; Kelly et al., 2001). Also polysaccharides and non-digestible oligosaccharides (inulin and other fructans, verbascose and other soybean oligosaccharides, lactulose, and others) are important in this respect, possibly by intervention in the composition of the microflora (Smits et al., 1996[a,b]; Buddington, 2001). Non-digestible oligosaccharides (NDO's) are characterized by being resistant to the intestinal enzymes of the host, but fermentable by bacteria (for instance *Lactobacilli* or *Bifidobacteria*) in the intestine (Buddington, 2001). Especially *Bifidobacteria* strongly proliferate after addition of NDO's to the diet (Gibson et al., 1995; Kleessen et al., 1997). Fermentation usually yields short chain fatty acids. NDO's may behave like prebiotics. Depending on structure and composition a NDO may be a preferential substrate for a specialized species or strain of bacteria. They may promote the relative proportions of that type of bacteria in the intestine, lower the pH and diminish the number of pathogens or putrefactive bacteria. In this respect the work of Houdijk (1998) may be of relevance. He studied the effect of two nondigestible oligosaccharides, fructooligosaccharides (FOS) and transgalactooligosaccharides (TOS), in weaner piglets and young pigs. No positive effects of FOS and TOS were observed on growth performance and apparent faecal and ileal nutrient digestion, though the pre-caecal digestibility of hemicellulose was enhanced. Of the FOS more than 90% was degraded pre-caecally. Some changes in fatty acid production were observed. More research is needed to clarify the effects of NDO's as prebiotics and to guide the choice for the most appropriate form of NDO for promoting intestinal health and function. Unfortunately, determination of changes in the composition of the intestinal flora has not been performed. Although promising as feed additives and growth promoters, caution is needed for too high doses, as osmotic diarrhea may be induced (Buddington, 2001).

Organic acids, especially the short chain fatty acids (SCFA), are important as determinants for intestinal mucosal growth and in the normal intestine they are mainly the anaerobic fermentation metabolites of the caecal and colonic resident microflora (Rowe et al., 1992; Sakata et al., 2001). SCFA in the hindgut increase the mucosal tissue mass of the large intestine as well as that of the small intestine. It is likely that the effect of SCFA on the small intestine is mediated by a systemic mediatory mechanism (Sakata et al., 2001). Short chain fatty acids like formiate, propionate and butyrate represent promising feed additives to replace the antibiotics. Recent experiments have demonstrated that after addition of organic acids to the diet the pH in the gut lumen was lowered upto the mid-jejunum (Mroz, personal communication). Although short chain fatty acids are known to be non-injurious preservatives (Moneret-Vautrin, 1986), their increasing consumption that creates a new micro-environment in the gut may interfere with gut homeostasis. In addition, agents that are physiologically relevant for the colonic epithelium may alter the process of cell proliferation. In studying physiologically relevant aspects of short chain fatty acids it was demonstrated in Caco-2 cell lines that butyrate induced a concentration dependent reversible increase in transepithelial electrical resistance (Mariadason et al., 1997). Moreover, the effect of butyrate paralleled changes in cellular differentiation. The specific activity of alkaline phosphatase was significantly increased.

Enterocytes are often studied in *in vitro* models such as the Caco-2 cells, that are derived from human colon adenocarcinoma (Pinto et al., 1983; Koninkx, 1995, see also the paragraph "Rationale justifying the use of Caco-2 cells in intestinal research"). In a recent experiment we have examined the effect of physiologically relevant concentrations of butyrate on Caco-2 cell proliferation by counting the number of cells at different time points. Except for 16 hours during which cells get attached to the surface, enterocyte-like Caco-2 cells were grown in cell culture medium containing 0, 1, 2, and 10 mM butyrate. A concentration dependent effect of butyrate on cell proliferation could be established (Table 2). Butyrate concentration of 2 mM had little or no effect at all on Caco-2 cell proliferation, whereas a high dose of 10 mM strongly inhibited cell growth. If Caco-2 cells were exposed to 1 mM butyrate, cell proliferation was stimulated. In this case the number of differentiated Caco-2 cells in the stationary phase of the growth curve appeared to be significantly higher.

Table 2. Concentration dependent effect of butyrate on Caco-2 cell proliferation

Days	Cell number. 10^{-6}			
	0 mM butyrate	1 mM butyrate	2 mM butyrate	10 mM butyrate
0	0.04	0.04	0.04	0.04
2	0.06	0.06	0.05	0.06
5	0.23	0.26	0.20	0.04[b]
9	0.98	1.21[a]	1.01	0.03[b]
12	1.01	1.39[a]	1.05	0.02[b]
16	0.95	1.43[a]	0.94	0.01[b]
19	1.00	1.45[a]	0.76[b]	0.01[b]

The results are mean values of 3 different Caco-2 cell passages and each experiment was performed in quadruplicate. [a]Significantly stimulated or [b]inhibited as compared to the control growth curve (0 mM butyrate) (p < 0.05). (Unpublished results)

3.3.3. Lectin-mucosa interactions

Some effects of dietary components on metabolism and activities of brush border enzymes in the rat small intestine can be demonstrated in a model in which rats are experimentally exposed to *Phaseolus vulgaris* lectins (Pusztai et al., 1996). Lectins are essential plant constituents and, thus, also found in the diet (Pusztai, 1993). Unfortunately, at a relatively high dietary intake of some lectins, such as phytohaemagglutinin (PHA), the lectin from kidney bean (*Phaseolus vulgaris*), wheat germ (*Triticum vulgare*) agglutinin (WGA), soybean (*Glycine max*) agglutinin (SBA) and many others can have harmful effects on the intestine (Figure 5). Interestingly, they are much less deleterious for germfree rats. This indicates that not all of the effects of deleterious lectins are direct, but that to some extent intestinal bacteria mediate these effects. In animals harbouring a gut flora, most of the harmful effects of 1% PHA appear to be due to the extensive overgrowth of *Escherichia coli* (Pusztai et al., 1993). Avidly binding lectins induce hyperplastic growth, increased turnover (Bardocz et al., 1995; Banwell et al., 1993) and thereby immature cells on the villi. The epithelial membranes of these immature cells contain many freely available mannose residues thereby facilitating the adherence and colonisation of *Escherichia coli* and other type-1 fimbriated bacteria (Pusztai et al., 1993).

One of the best ways to establish whether orally administered lectins could have any negative effects on gut metabolism is to monitor the possible changes in the activity of brush border membrane enzymes (Pusztai et al., 1996). Therefore, to establish the effects of lectins on nutritional performance of rats and epithelial cells, activities of brush border enzymes were measured in the small intestine of rats. The rats weighing 80 grams were fed for 10 days on either a control diet or a control diet including 0.7%

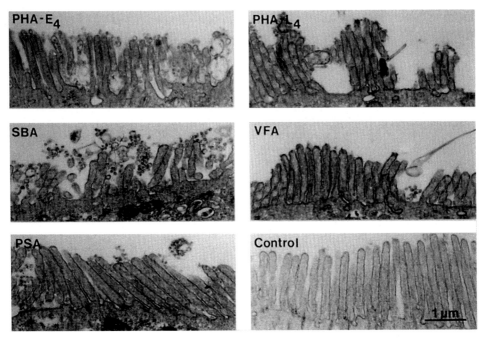

Figure 5. Damaged microvilli of differentiated Caco-2 cells after exposure to legume lectins.
Microvilli of Caco-2 cells incubated for 48 hours with 50 µg/ml each of PHA-E$_4$ (Phaseolus vulgaris isolectin E$_4$)(A), PHA-L$_4$ (Phaseolus vulgaris isolectin L$_4$) (B), SBA (Glycine max agglutinin) (C), Vicia faba agglutinin (VFA) (D), or Pisum sativum agglutinin (PSA) (E). The laesions diminish from A to E. Microvilli of control Caco-2 cells are present in (F). In legume exposed Caco-2 cells the presence of membrane-associated vesicles is obvious (bar = 1 µm).

GNA (*Galanthus nivalis* agglutinin, lectin of snowdrop bulbs) or 0.7% PHA as a toxic positive control. For comparison purposes GNA was selected in preference to others because, in preliminary studies with rats, it had only a slight effect on growth at dietary levels (Pusztai et al., 1990). At this level GNA had little or no effect at all on the weight and length of the small intestine (Table 3). Protein and DNA contents were slightly, but significantly, higher than in control rats.

The contrasting high increases in wet weight, length and DNA and protein contents of the small intestine induced by PHA-feeding further underlined the relatively low activity of GNA. However, the activities of brush border enzymes appeared to be affected. Total alkanine phosphatase activity of the entire small intestine of both GNA and PHA-fed rats was significantly higher than that of lactalbumin-fed control rats (table 3). Although the increase was slightly higher in GNA-fed rats than in the PHA group, the difference was not significant. Similarly, treatment with both GNA and PHA significantly elevated the total aminopeptidase activity of the rat small intestine. In this instance, the increase was more substantial with the PHA-fed rats and the

Table 3. Lectin-induced changes in growth, composition and digestive enzyme activities of the rat small intestine

	LA-fed	GNA-fed	PHA-fed	Pooled SD
Length (cm)	88.0	90.8[b]	106.7[a]	2.4
Wet weight (g)	4.7	4.5[b]	6.8[a]	0.4
Protein (mg)	322.0	401.0[a,b]	563.0[a]	31.1
DNA (mg)	23.3	29.0[a,b]	63.3[a]	4.8
Sucrase-isomaltase (U)	12.5	7.4[a]	6.9[a]	1.8
Alkaline phosphatase (U)	36.0	46.8[a]	43.4[a]	7.9
Aminopeptidase (U)	6.6	9.5[a,b]	12.2[a]	1.9

The results are mean values of length, wet weight, protein and DNA contents and mean activities of sucrase-isomaltase, alkaline phosphatase and aminopeptidase per small intestine of six rats. Pooled SD values were obtained by analysis of variance.
[a] Significantly different from lactalbumin (LA)-fed (control) rats ($p < 0.01$).
[b] Significantly different from PHA-fed rats ($p < 0.01$).
(After Pusztai et al., 1996)

difference between the two groups was significant. In contrast, the total mean sucrase-isomaltase activity of the small intestine of both GNA and PHA-fed rats was almost halved in comparison with controls. These effects are not due to bacterial overgrowth. Although most of the changes in gut metabolism caused by GNA in the diet were less extensive than those found with PHA, some of them may become potentially deleterious on longer exposure. Deleterious effects of lectins are due to binding to sugar components of glycoproteins. In the Caco-2 cell model it has been demonstrated that microvilli become disturbed by the mere presence of PHA (Koninkx et al., 1992). As expected also the enzyme activity of sucrase-isomaltase in differentiated Caco-2 cells decreased after exposure to PHA (recent unpublished results). These chains are strongly variable and therefore, it is not astonishing that effects in rats may be different from effects in piglets or chickens (Huisman et al., 1990; Simon, 2001).

As demonstrated above similar ligand-receptor interactions can be detrimental for enterocytes, but they also offer a scientific basis for a rational use of special components in diets to improve intestinal function (Naughton, 2001). Some of them may act as prebiotics (substances which stimulate and stabilise the health of the host by their effect on the intestinal microflora) by competing with unwanted micro-organisms for receptors or binding sites or they may activate advantageous intracellular pathways after binding to receptors. The same may apply for some probiotics (which are live micro-organisms with similar effects as prebiotics, for instance *Lactobacilli*, *Bifidobacteria*) (Huis in 't Veld et al., 1994; Morein et al., 2001).

3.3.4. Repair, defence, and resistance

Repair
Tight junctions connect the enterocytes to each other. They prevent macromolecular paracellular passage in a healthy intestine after weaning. Damage and leakage of tight junctions may permit paracellular passage of toxic, infectious and/or antigenic substances; in this way systemic effects, including food allergy, may result (Vellenga et al., 1985; Van Dijk et al., 1988; Stokes et al., 1997). If the mucosal barrier is really compromised, for instance by loss of (groups of) enterocytes, large amounts of macromolecules and even micro-organisms may invade the lamina propria and cause inflammatory responses.

Sometimes, deleterious agents are endocytosed by enterocytes, often after binding to a receptor on the surface of the cell. Mostly these phagosomes will fuse with lysosomes and killing of micro-organisms or degradation and hydrolysis by lysosomal enzymes will follow. A high activity of these enzymes is found in the differentiated enterocytes on the villi (Mouwen et al., 1983). However, some bacteria (such as *Salmonella, Listeria, Campylobacter, Mycobacterium*) may survive inside the enterocytes, largely hidden for defence mechanisms.

When the continuity of enterocytes is lost by death of (groups of) enterocytes the cells of the epithelial layer quickly restore the continuity by migration from the adjacent areas, gliding over the basal membrane which supports the epithelial cells. This process is called restitution. It can re-establish continuity within minutes to hours. To restore larger defects proliferation of epithelial cells is needed. This will start 12 to 16 hours after injury and after one to several days the missing epithelial cells will be replaced completely. Transforming growth factor ß, produced by wounded layers of intestinal epithelial cells, and polyamines appear to be the key molecules for restitution whereas transforming growth factor (is a strong promoter for proliferation. Many other peptide growth factors, such as trefoil peptides from the goblet cells and polyamines, may be involved in modulation of these processes (Bardócz et al., 1995; Göke et al., 1996; Koninkx et al., 1996). From this regulation of restitution and proliferation it is obvious that intestinal epithelial cells are able to synthesise cytokines, and as a matter of fact these cells can express the proteins or the mRNA's of many cytokines and cytokine receptors. Colostrum and milk contain many growth factors, including epidermal growth factor (EGF), insulin and insulin-like growth factors (IGF's), transforming growth factors (TGF's), colony stimulating factors, somatostatin, growth hormone, etc. Receptors for these polypeptides are present on enterocytes, especially in neonates but also in older animals. Most of them will remain biologically active during the intestinal transit, if milk proteins (casein) are present (Kelly et al., 1997).

Defence
In addition to growth promoting cytokines, enterocytes can synthesise bactericidal defensins and pro-inflammatory cytokines. For example, attachment of *Salmonella typhimurium* and enteroaggregative *Escherichia coli* (EAEC) to epithelial cells induces release of interleukin-8 (IL8) and other IL's (Gewirtz et al., 2000). It has been shown that after bacterial uptake by intestinal epithelial cells or active bacterial invasion of

these cells (Figure 6), pro-inflammatory cytokines and its mRNA's are very rapidly expressed by cultured intestinal cell lines or by freshly isolated intestinal cells. In this way interleukin-8, tumour necrosis factor-α, monocyte chemotactic factor-1 and granulocyte-macrophage colony-stimulating factor are secreted from the basolateral surface of the cells, facing the underlying tissues, and granulocytes and monocytes/macrophages are attracted and activated. After experimental infection it has been shown that inflammatory cells accumulate in close proximity of epithelial cells that are invaded by *Listeria* or *Salmonella* bacteria, as if they are waiting to

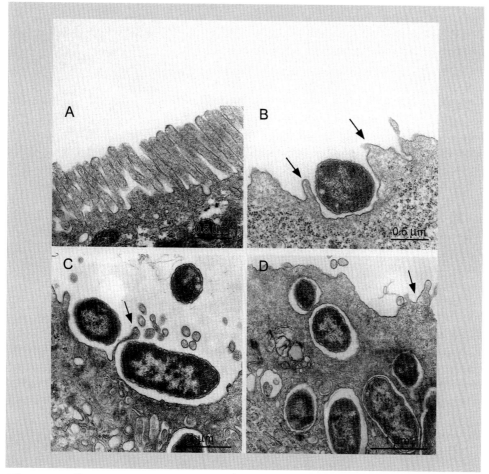

Figure 6. Adherence to and invasion of differentiated Caco-2 cells by Salmonella eneritidis.
Cells grown on tissue culture inserts (pore size 0.4 μm; growth area 1 cm^2) were incubated for 0 (A)(control), 10 (B), or 60 (C, and D) minutes with 1 ml of plain serum- and gentamicin-free cell culture medium containing 10^8 bacteria (200 bacteria/Caco-2 cell). Arrows indicate the presence of membrane ruffles (bar = 0.5 or 1 μm, respectively).

phagocytose the bacteria immediately after release from the epithelial cells. Only apical attachment of bacteria to cells of the small intestine did not evoke these responses, neither did bacterial lipopolysaccharide (Eckmann et al., 1995; own observations). The microbial/mucosal crosstalk between intestinal microflora and enterocytes may contribute significantly to prepare an adequate defence and to colonisation resistance (Kelly et al., 2001).

In addition to the first line of defence, as it is described above, a second line of defence exists. It forms a less circumscribed entity than the first one. A major part of it is the intestinal immune system and part of this system is concentrated in the gut associated lymphoid tissue (GALT), in the small intestine known as Peyer's patches. B and T cell areas, germinal centres and a specialised intestinal epithelium overlying the lymphoid dome, are essential components. In another chapter the intestinal immune system will be discussed in more detail by Goddeeris *cum suis*.

Resistance

Optimal quality of the barrier function of the intestinal epithelium, i.e. the mucus layer, the glycocalyx and the enterocytes, may warrant an optimal first line of resistance and defence. The genetics of the host and the intestinal micro-environment with its complex microbial flora will determine this quality (Morein et al., 2001; Kelly et al., 2001). However, the composition of this protective flora can be altered by dietary and environmental influences, making the host susceptible to disease. Probiotics are live microbial feed supplements which beneficially affect the host by improving the intestinal microbial balance (Fuller, 1989). Several modes of action are known which accomplish the beneficial effects of probiotics. One is the prevention of pathogen colonisation by competition for adhesion sites on the gut epithelial surface. Several lactic acid bacteria have been shown to be effective competitors, able to prevent adhesion of pathogens to intestinal cells (Jin et al., 1996) or to mucus (Ouwehand et al., 1996).

We have recently investigated the probiotic effect of two *Lactobacillus* strains on the sucrase-isomaltase activity in rat small intestine (Table 4). In all infected rats, irrespective of the bacteria used, the sucrase-isomaltase activity was significantly lower in comparison with control rats ($p < 0.01$). With respect to sucrase-isomaltase activity the beneficial effect of *Lactobacillus casei* and *Lactobacillus plantarum* could not be demonstrated. The difference in enzyme activity between *Salmonella enteritidis* infected rats and rats simultaneously infected with *Lactobacilli* and *Salmonella enteritidis* was not significant.

To enhance their resistance enterocytes, like other cells, can synthesise heat shock proteins (HSP's), for instance HSP27, HSP60, HSP70, HSP90, and others (the number indicates the molecular weight in kiloDalton). Heat shock proteins are chaperone proteins that protect the proteins during synthesis and immediately there after from immediate proteolysis and care for the development of the right secondary and tertiary configuration (Lindquist, 1986). This activity is enhanced as a universal and non-specific response to adverse changes in their environment, which is commonly known as the heat shock or stress response. Apparently a defensive mechanism, the transient heat shock response is a complex phenomenon that is rapidly induced and protects the cells from irreversible injury by stabilising the

Table 4. Sucrase-isomaltase activity in the rat small intestine after oral administration of *Salmonella enteritidis, Lactobacillus casei, Lactobacillus plantarum,* and successive oral administration of both *Lactobacilli* and *Salmonella enteritidis*.

Oral infection of rats	Sucrase-isomaltase activity (mU/mg protein)
Control	83.5 ± 8.1
Salmonella enteritidis	46.4 ± 5.4
Lactobacillus casei	60.1 ± 8.1
Lactobacillus casei/Salmonella enteritidis	48.1 ± 6.2
Lactobacillus plantarum	54.9 ± 9.8
Lactobacillus plantarum/Salmonella enteritidis	44.8 ± 2.5

Oral administration of *Salmonella enteritidis* (daily dosage 10^9 bacteria) was performed for 2 days, whereas *Lactobacillus casei* or *Lactobacillus plantarum* (daily dosage 10^9 bacteria) were administered for 11 days. To determine the probiotic effect of *Lactobacilli* the rats were infected with *Salmonella enteritidis* after 9 days of pre-treatment with *Lactobacilli*. On day 10 and 11 the rats were simultaneously infected with *Lactobacilli* and *Salmonella enteritidis*.
(Unpublished results)

synthetic and metabolic activities in the cell. The stress response is elicited by a variety of physical, chemical and microbiological agents, including heat shock, oxidising agents, heavy metals, sulphydryl reagents, anoxia, ethanol and various microorganisms. The most obvious characteristics of the stress response are an enhanced synthesis of heat shock proteins and a concomitant inhibition of overall protein synthesis. The heat shock proteins enable the cell to survive during stress and promote the resumption of normal cellular activities in the recovery period after stress. The enterocytes of the intestinal epithelium are regularly exposed to potentially harmful substances of dietary origin, such as lectins and bacteria. This results in a constant challenge of the intestinal cells. To withstand tissue damage the gut has evolutionary developed adaptive features to maintain its morphological and functional integrity and this tissue would benefit from high constitutive levels of heat shock proteins. The expression of heat shock proteins by this epithelium may be part of a protective mechanism developed by the intestinal cells to deal with noxious components in the intestinal lumen (Ovelgönne et al., 2000). In differentiated Caco-2 cells and rat jejunal epithelium we could clearly demonstrate that constitutive levels of heat shock proteins are present. The content of heat shock proteins of differentiated Caco-2 cells decreased in time during exposure to PHA-E$_4$ and WGA (Ovelgönne et al., 2000). This of course suggests that heat shock proteins are consumed in repairing sublethal cell damage without being adequately replenished. However, it appeared that the heat shock response was not impaired. Differentiated Caco-2 cells, pre-incubated with PHA-E$_4$ and WGA, were still capable of synthesising heat shock proteins after heat treatment (42^{0}C). In addition to damaging the apical membranes of the intestinal cells, depression of the heat shock protein synthesis in enterocytes by these lectins may leave the cells more vulnerable to exposure to harmful agents of dietary origin. Considering that pathogenic bacteria such as *Salmonella enteritidis* induce stress proteins in intestinal cells, lectin induced down-regulation of these proteins may also indicate increased cellular susceptibility to bacterial invasion.

In a recent study it has been clearly demonstrated that *Salmonella enteritidis*, which causes structural lesions and changes the mucosal integrity of differentiated Caco-2 cells on exposure, interferes with the levels of heat shock proteins 70 and 90 in these cells (Koninkx et al., 1999). *Salmonella enteritidis* significantly increases the levels of these heat shock proteins. The constitutive levels of heat shock proteins in the cells are obviously insufficient to protect the cells from invasion by bacteria. Even the increase in heat shock proteins induced by bacterial exposure did not protect the cells. However, such protection may be developed too late. To withstand tissue damage by bacteria and to immediately cope with this damage, cells would most likely benefit from previously induced high levels of heat shock proteins. Of course, synthesis of heat shock proteins is energy- and substrate consuming. However, the resistance to pathogens will be improved. If an additive (such as pre- and probiotics or short chain fatty acids) could increase the levels of heat shock proteins in enterocytes, it would provide these enterocytes with additional protection.

3.3.5. Recommendations for the use of parameters and techniques in pathological research

Many techniques and models for intestinal research have been discussed. A number of these parameters is still in process of development and needs to be validated. However, to our opinion a number of these models and techniques is already sufficiently validated and has enough potential impact to be used.

For morphological observation and examination of the integrity of the gut mucosa, and as indication for its normal functional potency, we recommend the measurements of length of the intestine and, microscopically, the villus height and crypt depth. From these data we calculate the villus/crypt ratio that informs us about the mucosal function as far as it is related to the quantitative parameter of surface. It is important to add information about the quality and maturity of the enterocytes. Immature cells on the villi may cause a weak barrier and they have impaired digestive and absorptive capacities. Therefore, villus and crypt measurements should be supported by one or more measurements of the activities of mucosal enzymes (we prefer sucrase-isomaltase, aminopeptidase and alkaline phosphatase), the number and quality of goblet cells (neutral, acid, sialo- and sulphomucins) or mucus analysis in intestinal chyme. High mitotic activity indicates fast renewal of enterocytes, resulting in immaturity. Influences of nutritional components on synthesis of DNA, RNA, and (glyco)proteins in intestinal epithelial cells can be determined (preferably *in vitro*) by incorporation of radioactive precursors in these cells. For an adequate interpretation of parameters related to digestive or absorptive capacity of the (small) intestine these parameters should not only be expressed as activity per weight or length unit of intestine, but as activity of the entire (small) intestine.

In addition, measurements of paracellular and transcellular permeability of parts of the intestine using the Ussing chamber technique offer significant parameters on intestinal function. Finally, demonstration of the presence of bacteria (or orally administered macromolecules) in lymph nodes or liver indicates translocation and impairment of the mucosal integrity, *i.e.* loss of barrier function.

Techniques to monitor the intestinal health as far as immunity and microflora are involvedare beyond the scope of this chapter.

3.3.6. Rationale justifying the in vitro use of cultured enterocytes in intestinal research

For *in vitro* culture of enterocytes, the cell lines Caco-2, HT-29 and HT-29 5M21 are often used cells. However, to compare *in vitro* data to data obtained in *in vivo* models, further research is required. Nevertheless, as pointed out in many studies the Caco-2 cell line derived from a human colon adenocarcinoma, is a unique *in vitro* model that is phenotypically similar to small intestinal cells (Pinto et al., 1983; Koninkx, 1995). This cell culture displays polarised enterocyte-like differentiation without synthesis of mucus. It is a suitable model to study general effects of, for instance, lectins (Draaier et al., 1989; Hendriks et al., 1991; Koninkx et al., 1992; Koninkx et al., 1996; Ovelgönne et al., 2000), short chain fatty acids (Basson et al., 1998; Schroder et al., 1999), pathogenic bacteria (Koninkx et al., 1999; Finley et al., 1990) and probiotics (Tuomola et al., 1998) at the cellular level. Undifferentiated Caco-2 cells can be regarded as an *in vitro* counterpart for immature crypt enterocytes, whereas the differentiated cells, exhibiting structural and functional properties of small intestinal enterocytes, may represent the *in vitro* counterpart for mature villus enterocytes (Table 5).

Growth and metabolic activity are monitored by measuring the synthesis of DNA, RNA and glycoprotein (incorporation of radioactive precursors). Functionality of the enterocytes is determined by measuring enzyme activities (sucrase-isomaltase, aminopeptidase, alkaline phosphatase). Sucrase-isomaltase is a marker enzyme that

Table 5. *In vivo* and *in vitro* models in intestinal research.

In vivo	In vitro
Animals	Caco-2 cells
Crypt cells • Undifferentiated • Cell growth/Cell proliferation	5-day old cells • Undifferentiated • Cell growth/Cell proliferation
Villus cells • Fully differentiated • No cell growth/cell proliferation	19-day old cells • Fully differentiated • No cell growth/cell proliferation

demonstrates the extent of differentiation of enterocytes; it is mainly present in the brush border membrane of villus cells and (almost) absent in crypt cells. This enzyme is involved in the terminal digestion of carbohydrates.

The quality and permeability of the tight junctions is reflected by the transepithelial electrical resistance (TEER) of monolayers of Caco-2 cells grown on filters (Figure 7). Culture on filters enables the division of the culture medium in an apical and a basolateral compartment (Figure 8). Increased permeability by leakage through the epithelial monolayer can be measured and may reflect the increased permeability as measured in the Ussing chamber model, or in *in vivo* models using indigestible high molecular compounds. However, further studies on this correlation are considered necessary. Modulating agents, such as dietary components, invading or non-invading bacteria or drugs can be offered at the apical or at the basolateral side of the enterocyte. Apical or basolateral secretion of cellular products or presence of mRNA's or proteins in the cell can be measured.

The morphological and functional characteristics of the HT-29 cell line, that is derived from a human colon adenocarcinoma, are very much the same as for the Caco-2 cell line. Through growth adaptation to methotrexate of the HT-29 cell line two new subclones have been isolated (Lesuffleur et al., 1990). The HT-29 5M12 subclone

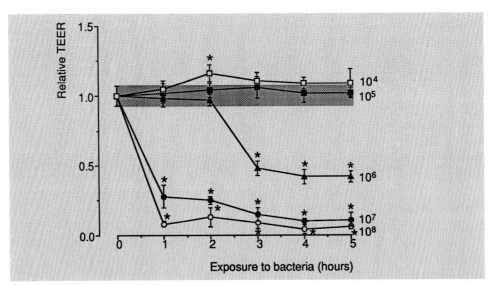

Figure 7. Dose-dependency of Salmonella enteritidis induced changes of the transepithelial electrical resistance (TEER) in monolayers of differentiated Caco-2 cells after apical exposure.

After exposure to Salmonella enteritidis (10^4, 10^5, 10^6, 10^7, and 10^8 bacteria/ml) for one hour changes in TEER were measured after 1, 2, 3, 4, and 5 hours). The results are expressed as the mean relative TEER ± SD. The dotted area represents the mean relative TEER ± SD of cell culture not exposed to bacteria. Significant differences (p < 0.05) between the relative levels of TEER of bacteria exposed and control cells have been indicated by an asterisk.

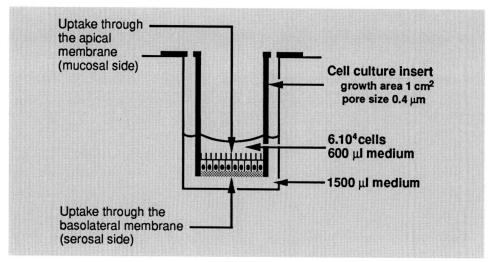

Figure 8. Schematic outline of the micoporous filter inserts used in uptake, transport and transepithelial electrical resistance studies of filter-grown differentiated Caco-2 cells.

Polarised enterocyte-like Caco-2 cells grown on a permeable filter (dotted area) mimic the *in vivo* animal model closely. Uptake and transport of (macro)molecules can be investigated from the apical (mucosal) compartment to the basolateral (serosal) compartment as well as in the opposite direction.

differentiates into columnar absorptive cells (enterocytes) and the HT-29 5M21 subclone into mucus-secreting goblet-like cells. This mucus-secreting subclone produces a mucus layer, which covers the cell surface of the entire cell monolayer, and is therefore more related to the *in vivo* situation, in which the mucus layer represents the first barrier to be taken by pathogens.

In our laboratory these models offer a relatively cheap, standardised and reproducible system with very limited variation, that is highly appropriate in detecting relatively small changes in cellular function and in establishing working mechanisms. Sometimes it has appeared to be appropriate to use additional cell lines with partially different enterocytic characteristics, such as the above-mentioned HT-29 subclones, with or without synthesis of mucus. However, function of the gut is more than just function of enterocytes. The interaction between enterocytes and the immune, endocrine or nervous system can not be studied in these *in vitro* models. Biopsies in organ culture seem to be an intermediate step between *in vitro* and animal models. However, from a morphological point of view the validity of results obtained in such systems is subject to debate. Even if the cells in these explants are still metabolically active, the morphological alterations are already severe after a short time of incubation. In our hands culture of explants during 5 hours appeared to be suitable to study pathological effects in enterocytes (Kik et al., 1991). The long distance for diffusion and the lack of circulation may be responsible for accumulation of metabolites, and deficiencies in oxygen and nutrients.

Even more than in germ free animals results based on experiments in *in vitro* models always need to be confirmed in studies with specified pathogen free or conventional animals and, eventually, in the target species in a field study. However, from a scientific and economical point of view the use of an *in vitro* model offers great advantages. These models enable great reduction of environmental influences on the experimental outcome, resulting in a better reproducibility and earlier detection of mechanisms with statistical significance. Relatively low costs and reduction of experimental animals are additional and important further advantages.

3.4. References

Banwell, J.G., R. Howard, I. Kabir, T.E. Adrian, R.H. Diamond, C. Abramowsky, 1993. Small intestinal growth caused by feeding red kidney bean phytohaemagglutinin lectin to rats. Gastroenterology 104, 1669-1677.

Bardocz, S., G. Grant, S.W.B. Ewen, T.J. Duguid, D.S. Brown, K. Englyst, A. Pusztai., 1995. Reversible effect of phytohaemagglutinin on the growth and metabolism of rat gastrointestinal tract. Gut 37, 353-360.

Bardócz, S., T.J.I. Duguid, D.S. Brown, G. Grant, A. Pusztai, A. White, A. Ralph, 1995. The importance of dietary polyamines in cell regeneration and growth. Brit. J. Nutr. 73, 819-828.

Basson, M.D., N.J. Emenaker, F. Hong, 1998. Differential modulation of human (Caco-2) colon cancer cell line phenotype by short chain fatty acids. Proc. Soc. Exper. Biol. Medic. 217, 476-483.

Buddington, R.K., 1997. Intestinal nutrient transport during the life history of swine. In: J.-P. Laplace, C. Février, A. Barbeau (Eds.), Digestive physiology in pigs. EAAP Publication No. 88, pp. 103-112.

Buddington, R.K., 2001. The use of nondigestible oligosaccharides to manage the gastrointestinal ecosystem. In: A. Piva, K.E. Bach Knudsen, J.E. Lindberg (Eds.), Gut environment of pigs. Nottingham University Press, Nottingham, United Kingdom, pp. 133-147.

Cranwell, P.D., 1995. Development of the gut and enzyme systems. In: M.A. Varley (Ed.), The neonatal pig: Development and survival. CAB International, Wallingford, United Kingdom, pp. 99-154.

Draaier, M., J. Koninkx, H. Hendriks, M. Kik, J. van Dijk, J. Mouwen, 1989. Actin cytoskeletal lesions in differentiated human colon carcinoma Caco-2 cells after exposure to soybean agglutinin. Biol. Cell 65, 29-35.

Eckmann, L., M.F. Kagnoff, J. Fieren, 1995. Intestinal epithelial cells as watchdogs for the natural immune system. Trends Microbiol. 3, 118-120.

Egberts, H.J.A., J.F.J.G. Koninkx, J.E. van Dijk, J.M.V.M. Mouwen, 1984. Biological and pathobiological aspects of the glycocalyx of the small intestinal epithelium. A review. Vet. Quart. 6, 35-48.

Ehsanullah, M., M.I. Filipe, B. Gazzard, 1982. Mucin secretion in inflammatory bowel disease: correlation with disease activity and dysplasia. Gut 23, 485-489.

Ferguson, A., E.E.E. Jarrett, 1975. Hypersensitivity reactions in the small intestine. 1. Thymus dependence of experimental "partial villous atrophy". Gut 16, 114-117.

Fernandez, F., R. Sharma, M. Bedford, 2000. Diet influences the colonisation of Campylobacter jejuni and distribution of mucin carbohydrates in the chick intestinal tract. Cell. Mol. Life Sci. 57, 1793-1801.

Filipe, M.I., C. Fenger, 1979. Histochemical characteristics of mucins in the small intestine. A comparative study of normal mucosa, benign epithelial tumours and carcinoma. Histochem. J. 11, 277-287.

Finlay, B.B., S. Falkow, 1990. Salmonella interacts with polarised human intestinal Caco-2 epithelial cells. J. Infect. Dis. 162, 1096-1106.

Forstner, G., A. Wesley, J. Forstner, 1982. Clinical aspects of gastrointestinal mucus. In: E.N. Chantler, J.B. Elder, M. Elstein (Eds.), Advances in Experimental Medicine and Biology. Plenum Press, New York, pp. 199-224.

Fuller, R., 1989. A review: Probiotics in man and animals. J. Appl. Bacteriol. 66, 365-378.

Gewirtz, A.T., A.S. Rao, P.O. Simon, D. Merlin, D. Carnes, J.L. Madara, A.S. Neish, 2000. Salmonella typhimurium induces epithelial IL8 expression via Ca^{2+}-mediated activation of the NF-κB pathway. J. Clin. Invest. 105, 79-92.

Gibson, G.R., Beatty, E.R., Wang, X., Cummings, J.H., 1995. Selective stimulation of Bifidobacteria in the human colon by oligofructose and inulin. Gastroenterol. 108, 975-982.

Göke, M, D.K. Podolsky, 1996. Regulation of the mucosal epithelial barrier. Baillieres Clin. Gastroenterol. 10: 393-405.

Hendriks, H.G.C.J.M., M.J.L. Kik, J.F.J.G. Koninkx, T.S.G.A.M. van den Ingh, J.M.V.M. Mouwen, 1991. Binding of kidney bean (Phaseolus vulgaris) isolectins to differentiated human colon carcinoma Caco-2 cells and their effect on cellular metabolism. Gut 32, 196-201.

Houdijk, J.G.M., 1998. Effects of non-digestible oligosaccharides in yong pig diets. PhD Thesis, Wageningen Agricultural University.

Huis in 't Veld, J.H.J., R. Havenaar, Ph. Marteau, 1994. Establishing a scientific basis for probiotic R&D. Tibtech. 12, 6-8.

Huisman, J., A.F.B. van der Poel, J.M.V.M. Mouwen, E.J. van Weerden, 1990. Effect of variable protein content in diets containing Phaseolus vulgaris beans on performance, organ weight and blood variables in piglets, rats and chickens. Br. J. Nutr. 64, 755-764.

Jin, L.Z., Y.W. Ho, M.A. Ali, N. Abdullah, S. Jalaludin, 1996. Effect of adherent Lactobacillus spp on the in vitro adherence of salmonellae to the intestinal epithelial cells of chicken. J. Appl. Bacteriol. 81, 201-206.

Kelly, D., A.P.G. Coutts, 1997. Biologically active peptides in colostrum and milk. In: J.-P. Laplace, C. Février, A. Barbeau (Eds.), Digestive physiology in pigs. EAAP Publication No. 88, pp. 163-170.

Kelly, D., T.P. King, 2001. Luminal bacteria:regulation of gut function and immunity. In: A. Piva, K.E. Bach Knudsen, J.E. Lindberg (Eds.), Gut environment of pigs. Nottingham University Press, Nottingham, United Kingdom, pp. 113-131.

Kik, M.J.L., J.F.J.G.Koninkx, A. van den Muysenberg, F. Hendriksen, 1991. Pathological effects of Phaseolus vulgaris isolectins in pig jejunal mucosa in organ culture. Gut 32, 886-892.

Kleessen, B., Sykura, B., Zunft, H.-J., Blaut, M., 1997. Effects of inulin and lactose on faecal microflora, microbial activity, and bowel habit in elderly constipated persons. Am. J. Clin. Nutr. 65, 1397-1402.

Koninkx, J., J. Swennenhuis, N. Nauta, H. Ovelgönne, H. Hendriks, W. Kok, J. van Dijk, 1999. Heat shock protein synthesis in enterocyte-like Caco-2 cells after exposure to bacteria. In: Å. Krogdahl, S.D. Mathieson, I.F. Pryme (Eds.), COST 98: Effects of Antinutrients on the Nutritional Value of Legume Diets (volume 8). Brussels, EU Publications pp. 38-43.

Koninkx, J.F.J.G., A.F.E. Stemerdink, M.H. Mirck, H.J.A. Egberts, J.E. van Dijk, J.M.V.M. Mouwen, 1988b. Histochemical changes in the composition of mucins in goblet cells during methotrexate-induced mucosal atrophy in rats. Exp. Pathol. 34, 125-133.

Koninkx, J.F.J.G., D.S. Brown, W. Kok, H.G.C.J.M. Hendriks, A. Pusztai, S. Bardocz, 1996. Polyamine metabolism of enterocyte-like Caco-2 cells after exposure to Phaseolus vulgaris lectin. Gut 38, 47-52.

Koninkx, J.F.J.G., H.G.C.J.M. Hendriks, J.M.A. van Rossum, T.S.G.A.M. van den Ingh, J.M.V.M. Mouwen, 1992. Interaction of legume lectins with the cellular metabolism of differentiated Caco-2 cells. Gastroenterology 102, 1516-1523.

Koninkx, J.F.J.G., M.H. Mirck, H.G.C.J.M. Hendriks, J.M.V.M. Mouwen, J.E. van Dijk, 1988. *Nippostrongylus brasiliensis*: Histochemical changes in the composition of mucins in goblet cells during infection in rats. Exp. Parasit. 65, 84-90.

Koninkx, J.F.J.G., 1995. Enterocyte-like Caco-2 cells as a tool to study lectin interaction. In: A. Pusztai, S. Bardocz (Eds.), Lectins: Biomedical Perspectives. Taylor and Francis, London, pp. 81-101.

Lamont, J.Th.,1992. Mucus: the front line of intestinal mucosal defense. Ann. N. Y. Acad. Sci. 664: 190-201.

Lesuffleur, T., Barbat, A., Dussaulx, E., Zweibaum, A. 1990. Growth adaptation to methotrexate of HT-29 colon carcinoma cells is associated with their ability to differentiate into columnar absorptive and mucus-secreting cells. Cancer Res. 40: 6334-6343.

Lindquist, S., 1986. The heat shock response. Ann. Rev. Biochem. 55, 1151-1191.

Mantle, M., A. Allen, 1989. Gastrointestinal mucus. In: J.S. Davison (Ed.), Gastrointestinal secretion. University Press, London, pp. 202-229.

Mariadason, J.M., D.H. Barkla, P.R. Gibson, 1997. Effect of short chain fatty acids on paracellular permeability in Caco-2 intestinal epithelium model. Am. J. Physiol. 272, G705-G712.

McCracken, B.A., Gaskins, H.R., Ruwe-Kaiser, P.J., Klasing, K.C., Jewel, D.E., 1995. Diet-dependent and diet-independent metabolic responses underlie growth stasis of pigs at weaning. J. Nutr. 125, 2838-2845.

Moneret-Vautrin, D.A., 1986. Food antigens and additives. J. Allergy Clin. Immunol. 78, 1039-1044.

Morein, B., Ke-Fei Hu, 2001. Microorganisms exert bioactive and protective effects through the innate immune system. In: A. Piva, K.E. Bach Knudsen, J.E. Lindberg (Eds.), Gut environment of pigs. Nottingham University Press, Nottingham, United Kingdom, pp. 105-111.

Mouwen, J.M.V.M., H.J.A. Egberts, J.F.J.G. Koninkx, 1983. The outermost mucosal barrier of the mammalian small intestine. Dtsch. Tierärztl. Wschr. 90, 477-482.

Naughton, P.J., 2001. Lectin microbial interactions in the gut. In: A. Piva, K.E. Bach Knudsen, J.E. Lindberg (Eds.), Gut environment of pigs. Nottingham University Press, Nottingham, United Kingdom, pp. 149-163.

Ouwehand, A.C., P.L. Conway, 1996. Purification and characterisation of a component produced by Lactobacillus fermentum that inhibits the adhesion of K88 expressing Escherichia coli to porcine ileal mucus. J. Appl. Bacteriol. 80, 311-318.

Ovelgönne, J.H., J.F.J.G. Koninkx, A. Pusztai, S. Bardocz, W. Kok, S.W.B. Ewen, H.G.C.J.M. Hendriks, J.E. van Dijk, 2000. Decreased levels of heat shock proteins in gut epithelial cells after exposure to plant lectins. Gut 46, 679-687.

Pinto, M., S. Robine-Leon, M.D. Appay, M. Kedinger, N. Triadou, E. Dussaulx, B. Lacroix, P. Simon-Assmann, K. Haffen, J. Fogh, A. Zweibaum, 1983. Enterocyte-like differentiation and polarisation of the human colon carcinoma cell line Caco-2 in culture. Biol. Cell 47, 323-330.

Pluske, J.R., 2001. Morphological and functional changes in the small intestine of the newly-weaned pig. In: A. Piva, K.E. Bach Knudsen, J.E. Lindberg (Eds.), Gut environment of pigs. Nottingham University Press, Nottingham, United Kingdom, pp. 1-27.

Puchal, A.A., R.K. Buddington, 1992. Postnatal development of monosaccharide transport in pig intestine. Am. J. Physiol. 262, G895-G902.

Pusztai A., 1993. Dietary lectins are metabolic signals for the gut and modulate immune and hormone functions. European Journal of Clinical Nutrition 47, 691-699.

Pusztai, A., G. Grant, R.J. Spencer, T.J. Duguid, D.S. Brown, S.W.B. Ewen, W.J. Peumans, E.J.M. Van Damme, S. Bardocz, 1995. Kidney bean lectin-induced Escherichia coli overgrowth in the small intestine is blocked by GNA, a mannose-specific lectin. Journal of Applied Bacteriology 75, 360-368.

Pusztai, A., J. Koninkx, H. Hendriks, W. Kok, S. Hulscher, E.J.M. Van Damme, W.J. Peumans, G. Grant, S. Bardocz, 1996. Effect of the insecticidal Galanthus nivalis agglutinin on metabolism and the activities of brush border enzymes in the rat small intestine. J. Nutr. Biochem. 7, 677-682.

Pusztai, A., S.W.B. Ewen, G. Grant, W.J. Peumans, E.J.M. Van Damme, L. Rubio, S. Bardocz, 1990. The relationship between survival and binding of plant lectins during small intestinal passage and their effectiveness as growth factors. Digestion 46, 308-316.

Reid, P.E., C.F.A. Culling, W.L. Dunn, M.G. Clay, 1984. Chemical and histochemical studies of normal and diseased human gastrointestinal tract. 2. A comparison between histochemically normal intestine and Crohn's disease of the small intestine. Histochem. J. 16, 253-264.

Rowe, W.A., T.M. Bayless, 1992. Colonic short chain fatty acids: fuel from the lumen? Gastroenterology 103, 336-337.

Sakata, T., A. Inagaki, 2001. Organic acid production in the large intestine: implication for epithelial cell proliferation and cell death. In: A. Piva, K.E. Bach Knudsen, J.E. Lindberg (Eds.), Gut environment of pigs. Nottingham University Press, Nottingham, United Kingdom, pp. 85-94.

Sangild, P.T., 1997. Peri-natal development of gut enzyme activity: intrinsic mechanisms versus external influences. In: J.-P. Laplace, C. Février, A. Barbeau (Eds.), Digestive physiology in pigs. EAAP Publication No. 88, pp. 118-126.

Sangild, P.T., 2001. Transitions in the life of the gut at birth. In: J.E. Lindberg and B. Ogle (Eds.), Digestive Physiology in Pigs. CABI Publishing, Wallingford (UK) / New York (USA), pp. 3-17.

Schroder, O., S. Hess, W.F. Caspary, J. Stein, 1999. Mediation of differentiating effects of butyrate on the intestinal cell line Caco-2 by transforming growth factor $\beta 1$. Eur. J. Nutr. 38, 45-50.

Simon, O., 2001. The influence of feed composition on protein metabolism in the gut. In: A. Piva, K.E. Bach Knudsen, J.E. Lindberg (Eds.), Gut environment of pigs. Nottingham University Press, Nottingham, United Kingdom, pp. 63-84.

Smith, M.W., 1988. Postnatal development of transport function in the pig intestine. Comp. Biochem. Physiol. 90A, 577-582.

Smits, C.H.M., C.A.A. te Maarsen, J.M.V.M. Mouwen, J.F.J.G. Koninkx, 1996[a]. The antinutritive effect of a carboxymethylcellulose with high viscosity in broiler chickens is not associated with mucosal damage. In: C.H.M. Smits, Viscosity of dietary fibre in relation to lipid digestibility in broiler chickens. Ph.D. Thesis, Wageningen Agricultural University, pp. 71-80.

Smits, C.H.M.,A.V. Veldman, M.W.A. Verstegen, A.C. Beynen, 1996[b]. Dietary carboxymethylcellulose with high instead of low viscosity reduces macronutrient digestion in broiler chickens. In: C.H.M. Smits, Viscosity of dietary fibre in relation to lipid digestibility in broiler chickens. Ph.D. Thesis, Wageningen Agricultural University, pp. 41-54.

Stokes, C.R., M. Bailey, K. Haverson, P.W. Bland, 1997. The role of the gastrointestinal immune system in the control of responses to dietary antigens. In: J.-P. Laplace, C. Février, A. Barbeau (Eds.), Digestive physiology in pigs. EAAP Publication No. 88, pp. 212-221.

Tuomola, E.M., S.J. Salminen, 1998. Adhesion of some probiotic and dairy Lactobacillus strains to Caco-2 cell cultures. Internat. J. Food Microbiol. 41, 45-51.

Turani, H., B. Lurie, C.H. Chaimoff, E. Kessler, 1986. The diagnostic significance of sulphated acid mucin content in gastric intestinal metaplasia with early gastric cancer. Am. J. Gastroenterol. 81, 343-345.

Van Beers-Schreurs, H.M.G., M.J.A. Nabuurs, L. Vellenga, H.J. Kalsbeek-van der Valk, T. Wensing, H.J. Breukink, 1998. Weaning and the weanling diet influence the villous height and crypt depth in the small intestine of pigs and alter concentrations of short-chain fatty acids in the large intestine and blood. J. Nutr. 128, 947-953.

Van der Klis, J.D., A. van der Voorst, 1993. The effect of carboxymethylcellulose (a soluble polysaccharide) on the rate of marker excretion from the gastrointestinal tract of broilers. Poultry Sci. 72, 503-512.

Van Dijk, A.J., 2001. Spray-dried animal plasma in the diet of piglets: Influence on growth performance and underlying mechanisms. Ph.D. Thesis, Utrecht University.

Van Dijk, A.J., Everts, H., Nabuurs, M.J.A., Margry, R.J.C.F., Beynen, A.C., 2001. Growth performance of weanling piglets fed spray-dried animal plasma: a review. Livest. Prod. Sci. 68, 263-274.

Van Dijk, J.E., A. Fledderus, J.M.V.M. Mouwen, C. Holzhauer, 1988. Gastrointestinal food allergy and its role in large domestic animals. Vet. Res. Comm. 12, 47-59.

Van Leeuwen, P., E. Esteve-Garcia, J.C. Meijer, F.G. van Zijderveld, J.M.V.M. Mouwen, and M.W.A. Verstegen, 2001. Effects of Virginiamycin, as feed additive, on histological parameters of the small intestinal mucosa and on performance in piglets (in preparation).

Vellenga, L., J.M.V.M. Mouwen, J.E. van Dijk, H.J. Breukink, 1985. Biological and pathological aspects of the mammalian small intestinal permeability to macromolecules. Vet. Quart. 7, 322-332.

Weström, B.R., 1997. The young pig as a model for intestinal absorption of macromolecules. In: J.-P. Laplace, C. Février, A. Barbeau (Eds.), Digestive physiology in pigs. EAAP Publication No. 88, pp. pp. 37-40.

Xu, R.J., D.J. Mellor, P. Tungthanathanich, M.J. Birtles, G.W. Reynolds, H.V. Simpson, 1992. Growth and morphological changes in the small intestine and the large intestine in piglets during the first three days after birth. J. Develop. Physiol. 18, 161-172.

4. The porcine and avian intestinal immune system and its nutritional modulation

B.M. Goddeeris[1,2], W.J.A. Boersma[3], E. Cox[1], Y. Van der Stede[1], M.E. Koenen[3], S. Vancaeneghem[1], J. Mast[4] and W. Van den Broeck[5]

[1] Department Virology Parasitology Immunology, Faculty of Veterinary Medicine, University of Gent, Salisburylaan 133, 9820 Merelbeke, Belgium. E-mail: bruno.goddeeris@agr.kuleuven.ac.be

[2] Laboratory for Physiology and Immunology, Departement of Animal Sciences, K.U.Leuven, Kardinaal Mercierlaan 92, 3001 Heverlee, Belgium

[3] Division Animal Science, Research Group Animal Physiology and Health, Institute for Animal Science and Health ID-Lelystad, PO Box 65, 8200 AB Lelystad, The Netherlands

[4] Department Biocontrol, CODA, Groeselenberg 99, 1180 Ukkel, Belgium

[5] Department of Morphology, Faculty of Veterinary Medicine, University of Gent, Salisburylaan 133, 9820 Merelbeke, Belgium.

Abstract

In order to comprehend the influence of nutrition on the immune system and responsiveness of poultry and swine, the immune system and in particular the gut-associated lymphoid tissue (GALT) and its components are reviewed. As nutritional factors act often on the induction phase of the immune response, attention is also focussed on the acute-phase response that is responsible for the ensuing immune and physiological reactions. Several methods that can be used to analyse the interaction of nutrition on the immune system are discussed.

In a second part we focussed on different feed manipulations that can alter immune responsiveness and paid special attention to our own research areas. Feed restriction, the ratio of n-3 to n-6 poly-unsaturated fatty acids in the feed, the inclusion of prebiotics such as vitamin D and A, β-glucans, carnitine, dietary nucleotides and finally the addition of probiotics are discussed to explain the influence of nutritional factors on the immune response and their way of action.

Keywords: GALT, immunomodulation, nutrition, β-glucans, probiotics, prebiotics

4.1. Introduction

For economical reasons, the poultry and pig industry is marked today by a phenotypic inbreeding for production parameters that might result in a genotypic linkage with an altered (compromised) immune responsiveness. A well-developed immune system and optimal immune responsiveness remain important for the welfare and productivity. Indeed these qualities can only be obtained if the health status of the animal scores high. Therefore a lot of energy and money is invested in prophylactic measures such as vaccinations and chemoprophylaxis against infectious diseases. However, health and immune responsiveness is not only maintained and improved by vaccinations and hygiene but also by an adequate supply of nutritional components to the animal. Moreover, immune reactivity and alertness of the gastrointestinal tract can be modulated (improved or oriented) by nutritional interventions such as feed restriction or alterations in minerals, vitamins, essential fatty acids or other substances. In order to modulate or influence the immune response or responsiveness of an animal by nutrition it is important to understand the basic immune effector mechanisms and factors influencing these. Therefore, a fundamental knowledge on the intricate communication of the immunocompetent cells, their induction sites (GALT), signals (cytokines) and in particular the acute phase response which is responsible for initiating immune responses, is required for understanding and improving dietary modulation of immune responsiveness.

4.2. The immunocompetent cells

4.2.1. The leukocytes

The immunocompetent cells can be divided in the antigen specific and a-specific cells. The antigen a-specific cells are responsible for the innate immunity, the first immune defence that occurs upon tissue alterations such as tissue damage, introduction of foreign antigen or invasion by pathogens. These cells play also an important role in the repair of tissue damage. However, their important immune role is not restricted to a first-line defence but lays also in the triggering of alarm signals which are crucial for initiating and directing subsequent antigen a-specific and specific defence reactions.

The antigen a-specific cells consist primarily of phagocytes, i.e. monocyte/macrophages, neutrophils (called heterophils in birds) and thrombocytes. *In vivo* and *in vitro* studies have shown that the latter are active phagocytes in the chicken (Chang and Hamilton, 1979). Monocytes emigrate from the bone marrow into the blood circulation to reach subsequently the tissues where they differentiate into resident macrophages. There they act for months as sentinels for changes and invaders. Neutrophils that have a shorter half-life (days) and are the first-line soldiers who die in battle, reach in a similar way the tissues in search for foreign invaders but do recirculate. However, as has been evidenced in mammals, an important number of neutrophils remains attached to the endothelium of the blood vessels where they detach in massive numbers upon receiving alarm signals such as fever and immune/endocrine signals that have been induced by alerted macrophages (sentinels).

Table 1. The orchestra: the antigen-specific and antigen-presenting (target) cells, their cell membrane molecules and their products.

Instruments (molecules)	Musicians (cells)		Music (products)
MHC class II	CD4 target cell	→ APC: IDC, macrophages, B cells	Cytokines
MHC class I	CD8 target cell	→ Infected cells, tumor cells	Death
TCR, CD4	CD4+ T cell	→ Helper T cell (Th1, Th2, Th3)	Cytokines, cytotoxins
TCR, CD8	CD8+ T cell	→ Cytotoxic T cell	Cytotoxins, granzymes, perforines
BCR	B cells	→ Plasma cells	Antibodies

The antigen specific cells are divided in two main populations: the B cells and the T cells. Their antigen specificity is mediated by cell surface receptors, the B cell receptor (membrane-bound immunoglobulin, BCR) and the T cell receptor (TCR), respectively (table1). The repertoire of each of these receptors for their different antigens is clonally distributed, i.e. each individual T cell and B cell has only one idiotypic set of antigen receptors and can thus only recognize one specific antigen (epitope). B cells recognize with their BCR directly a specific epitope of an unprocessed antigen. T cells on the other hand, recognize with their TCR epitopes of a processed antigen on the surface of an antigen-presenting cell. Indeed, the proteinaceous antigen is processed intracellularly by an antigen-presenting cell into linear epitopes of 10 to 20 amino

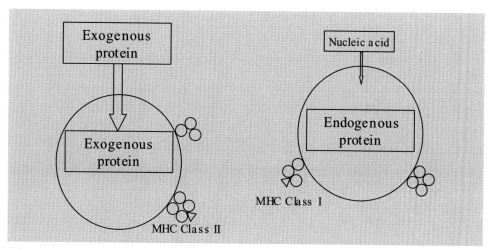

Figure 1. Presentation of processed antigens (peptides: T cell epitopes) of exogenous and endogenous antigens in association with MHC class II and MHC class I molecules, respectively.

acids long that associate intracellularly with major histocompatibility complex (MHC) molecules. These MHC molecules will, on subsequent expression on the cell membrane of the antigen-presenting cell, present the epitope to the T cell.

The T cell population can be subdivided in CD4+ and CD8+ T cells (in swine there exist also double positive and double negative T cells) (table 1). CD4+ T cells recognize their epitope in association with MHC class II molecules while CD8+ T cells recognize their epitope in association with MHC class I molecules (figure 1). MHC class II molecules present epitopes from exogenous antigens, i.e. phagosomal antigens which have been taken up by the antigen-presenting cell, while MHC class I molecules present epitopes from endogenous antigens, i.e. cytoplasmic antigens which have been transcribed inside the antigen-presenting cell as is the case in virus-infected cells. This difference has very important consequences as CD4+ T cells are helper T cells which deliver help to their antigen-presenting target cell by secretion of cytokines, while CD8+ T cells are cytotoxic T cells which kill their infected target cell by cytotoxic signal transduction and cytotoxic factors (figure 2, table 2).

In mice, two kind of helper T (Th) cells have been recognized based on their cytokine profiles: the Th1 is characterized by the secretion of interleukin-2 (IL-2), interferon-γ (IFN-γ) and tumor necrosis factor α (TNF-α) while the Th2 is characterized by IL-4, IL-5, IL-10 and transforming growth factor β (TGF-β). The latter cytokine is now claimed to be produced by a third T helper cell population, namely Th3. The type of cytokine(s) produced has important implications on the target cells e.g. it determines which antibody isotype will be produced by the activated B cell. Whether these types of helper T cells also exist in poultry is not yet known but evidence exists that at least some of these different cytokines are also present in birds and could thus influence the type of immune response induced.

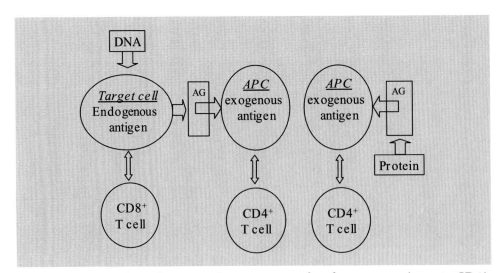

Figure 2. Presentation of processed exogenous and endogenous antigens to CD4+ and CD8+ T cells, respectively.

Table 2. The performance of the score: antigen-specific induction of an immune response

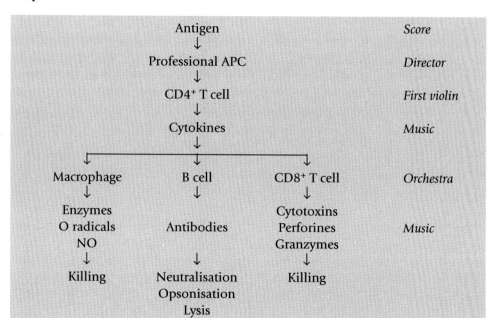

	Score
Antigen	
↓	
Professional APC	Director
↓	
CD4+ T cell	First violin
↓	
Cytokines	Music

Macrophage	B cell	CD8+ T cell	Orchestra
↓	↓	↓	
Enzymes O radicals NO	Antibodies	Cytotoxins Perforines Granzymes	Music
↓	↓	↓	
Killing	Neutralisation Opsonisation Lysis	Killing	

4.2.2. The secondary lymphoid structures: the induction site of B and T cells

Primary induction of immune responses occurs in the secondary lymphoid organs. These structures are filters for antigen (or antigen bearing APC) and naive lymphocytes and are optimally organized for intercellular communication between antigen-presenting cells, T cells and B cells. These organs are strategically placed on the lymph (lymph nodes) and blood circulation (spleen) to capture antigen and antigen-presenting cells draining from the tissues. By specific adhesion molecules, naive lymphocytes are directed to emigrate from the blood circulation into these secondary lymphoid organs in search for their specific antigen.

Compared to other mammals, the pig has an inverted structure of its lymph nodes with the medulla being external to the cortex. Nevertheless, the physiology of the T and B cell areas are broadly conventional, with the T cell zone located in the paracortex and the B cell zone with its follicles located in the cortex. T and B cells enter via paracortical postcapillary venules, of which many are high endothelial venules (HEV). The major difference between pigs and other mammals lies in the emigration route of the lymphocytes: instead of leaving by sinuses through the medulla in the afferent lymph, they emigrate directly into the blood through the HEV (Binns and Pabst, 1988; Pabst and Binns, 1989; Binns and Pabst, 1994). As a consequence, efferent lymph of pigs contains very few lymphoid cells as compared to other species. The porcine spleen is composed of white and red pulp. The white pulp contains mainly leukocytes while the red pulp consists of erythrocytes and lymphocytes. In the white pulp lymphocytes are organised around the arterioles in peri-arteriolar lymphoid sheets (PALS). The peri-arteriolar sheet consists of a mantel of T cells (CD4$^+$>CD8$^+$) surrounded by a marginal zone containing macrophages and B cells. T cells are also found in the red pulp (CD8$^+$>CD4$^+$) (Bianchi *et al.*, 1992). These cells are already present at birth, but a large increase occurs after 2 weeks of life. At the same time, a similar increase occurs in B cells, mainly IgM$^+$, with the formation of small follicles in the PALS as a consequence. In 4-week-old pigs the percentage of B cells in regard to the total amount of lymphoid cells, is similar to that in peripheral blood, approximately 35%. Most IgM-producing cells are located in the red pulp, whereas IgG- and IgA-producing cells are predominantly present in the periphery of the PALS (Bianchi *et al.*, 1992). At 10 months of age however, IgG and IgA-producing cells can also be found in the red pulp.

Peripheral lymph nodes appear to be absent in the chicken. The adult chicken spleen however is a well-organized organ that is composed of white and red pulp, consisting mainly of leukocytes and erythrocytes, respectively. The leukocytes in the white pulp are distributed in two structures, the peri-arteriolar lymphoid sheath (PALS) and the peri-ellipsoid lymphoid sheath (PELS). The PALS surrounds the arterioles of the spleen and is mainly composed of T cells while the PELS surrounds the sinusoids, bordered by the ellipsoid-associated reticular cells, and is mainly composed of resting B cells enclosed by a ring of macrophages (Mast and Goddeeris, 1998a,b). These resting B cells (PELS) are supposed to trap antigen coming from the sinusoids and to migrate subsequently to the T cell zone (PALS) where they can be activated and form germinal centres.

Early in the development of the chicken spleen, sub-populations of T cells, B cells and macrophages as well as reticular cells are detected. Nevertheless, the first elements of typical structural organization of the spleen as described above are only formed around ED20. The PALS (T cell compartment) and especially the PELS (B cell compartment) gradually mature during the first week post-hatch (Mast and Goddeeris, 1999). This implies, assuming a strong relationship between structural organization and function, that the immune function of the late embryonic and neonatal spleen is not entirely developed. Indeed, immunization experiments with non-replicating immunogens indicate that the chick is only able to generate an antigen specific antibody response from 1 week of age onwards (Mast and Goddeeris, 1999).

4.3. The gut mucosal defence mechanisms

4.3.1. Non-immunological mucosal defense

Non-immunological defence mechanisms at mucosal surfaces are as important as the immunologically based defence mechanisms in protecting animals against invaders. This is evidenced by the appearance of diseases when one of these non-immunological defences starts to fail. Conversely, some of the beneficial effects of probiotics (see later) are claimed to operate through these non-immunological defence mechanisms. The non-immunological defence encompasses the following elements:

- intestinal and mucosal cleaning by peristalsis which assures a continuous passage of the intestinal contents,
- production of stomach acid and bile salts which creates a mucosal environment unsuitable for the growth of pathogens,
- mucus production that limits the penetration of micro-organisms,
- continuous turnover of the gastrointestinal epithelium by growth, migration and exfoliation (removal) of epithelial cells from the crypts towards the tip of the villi,
- production of lactoferrin, lactoperoxidase and lysozymes that inhibit proliferation of micro-organisms
- presence of a residual bacterial microflora that co-inhibits colonization and growth of pathogens.

4.3.2. Immunological defence: the gut-associated lymphoid tissue (GALT)

The immune defence system consists of lymphoid tissues and cells distributed along the gastrointestinal tract. The lymphoid tissue localized along the gastrointestinal tract constitutes quantitatively the major part of the immune system of the whole body. This extremely developed gastrointestinal immune system reflects the importance of the mucosal immune defence system against the continuous attack of antigens and pathogens. Moreover, the major development of this local immune tissue seems to be induced by the continuous attack by pathogens as evidenced by the atrophic mucosal immune system of pathogen-free animals (see later in probiotics).
Some important features characterize the mucosal immune system:
- it possesses specialised structures such as the Peyer's patches (PP) where induction of immune responses happen,
- certain subpopulations of lymphoid cells predominate at the mucosal surfaces,
- there is a specific recirculation of mucosal lymphocytes towards mucosae, known as mucosal homing, and
- the predominant mucosal immunoglobuline is dimeric IgA which is secreted at the mucosal surface.

All these elements of the mucosal immune system are working together to generate immune responses that protect the host against mucosal invaders but also render the host tolerant against ubiquitous dietary antigens and the beneficial microbial flora of the mucosae. The elucidation of the mechanisms that determine immunotolerance or immunoinduction forms today a major topic of study.
The gastrointestinal immune system consists of lymphoid cells in organised sites like PP and mesenterial lymph nodes, and lymphocytes spread over the stromal tissues in the lamina propria and the epithelium (the intra-epithelial lymphocytes, IEL) of the intestine. This immune system associated with the gastrointestinal tract and the respiratory tract are referred to as the gut-associated lymphoid tissue (GALT) and bronchial associated lymphoid tissue (BALT), respectively.
There exists evidence that these organized structures are the places (or one of the places) where antigen enters the mucosal immune system to initiate subsequently the immune reactions: therefore these places are quite often called the inductive lymphoid sites of the mucosal immune system. Lymphocytes located in the lamina propria and between

the epithelial cells of the intestinal tract are attributed with an effector function, such as antibody production, cytokine production and cytotoxicity, and are therefore referred to as the effector sites of the intestinal tract. These inductive and effector sites are interconnected by selective migration of lymphocytes (homing) whereby cells that have been activated in the inductive sites migrate specifically to effector sites of the intestinal tract. This interconnection assures that mucosal responses are primarily directed and localised against antigens that have been recognized at mucosal surfaces.

The Peyer's patches of the pig
Peyer's patches are aggregates of lymphoid follicles. In the pig there are different separate categories of PP (Binns and Licence, 1985). The first kind of PP is distributed as discrete patches along the jejunum and proximal ileum (jejunal PP). There are approximately 25 to 35 of these patches, and they are relatively small and persist throughout life (Pabst *et al.*, 1988; Stokes *et al.*, 1994). The second kind of PP is a very large single ileal PP which may extend for up to 2.5 m along the terminal ileum but shrinks at about 1 year of age to become a series of isolated patches (Stokes *et al.*, 1994). Below the ileo-caecal junction are situated a third PP, the spiral colon PP and more distally, large numbers of single 2-3 mm patches (Binns and Pabst, 1988).

The jejunal and ileal PP consist of B follicles with interfollicular areas (IFA) of T cells between the different follicles, and a dome area between the follicles and the epithelium (Bianchi *et al.*, 1992) (figure 3). The domes are covered by the follicle-

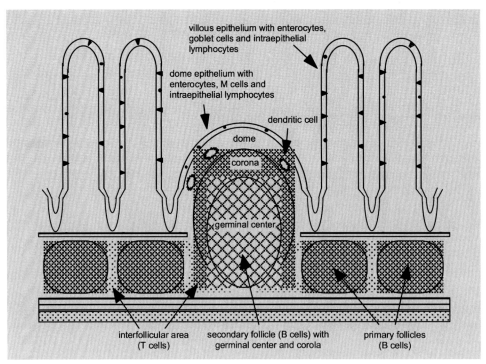

Figure 3. Schematic presentation of an ileal PP of the pig.

associated epithelium (FAE) while the IFA are covered by villi. The epithelium overlaying the dome consists of epithelial cells and M (microfold) cells which appear to play an important role in the uptake of particulate antigens. M cells have increased numbers of cytoplasmic vesicles in which particulate antigen is transported across the cell from the luminal to the basement membrane surface (Smith and Peacock, 1992). Consequently, the antigen is transported into the dome region of the PP where it is taken up by macrophages, dendritic cells and B cells, which process and present the antigen in a MHC class II-restricted way to local CD4$^+$ T cells (MacDonald and Carter, 1982). These activated T cells will then provide help to the B cells. Follicles with germinal centres are located under the dome. The proliferating B cells in that area consist mainly of IgA$^+$ B cells. However, these B cells undergo here no terminal differentiation but migrate via the lymph, mesenteric lymph nodes and finally the blood to distant places in the lamina propria, where they will undergo final differentiation into IgA-producing plasma cells.

The intestinal lamina propria of the pig
The intestinal lamina propria consists of a fibrous space between the muscularis mucosae and the epithelial cells. It contains capillaries that allow the extravasation of lymphoid cells. The lamina propria contains a lot of lymphocytes, plasma cells and macrophages. Also mast cells and eosinophils are here present. In newborn piglets, the T cells are more numerous in the crypts than in the villi, whereas in 6-month-old pigs, more T cells are found in the villi than in the crypts (Stokes *et al.*, 1994). During the first days of life T cells are mainly CD8$^+$, whereas CD4$^+$ T cells predominate from 14 days of age. In conventional adult swine, CD4$^+$ cells are thus more numerous than CD8$^+$ cells in the lamina propria, with the CD4$^+$ cells being compartmentalized in the core of the villi and the CD8$^+$ cells immediately below the epithelium (Vega-Lopez *et al.*, 1993) (figure 4). With respect to B cells during the first period of life, the IgM-producing cells outnumber the IgA-producing cells in the lamina propria, but the incidence of both are comparable from 5 weeks of age. IgG-producing cells are less present and not observed before two weeks of age. In 6-month-old pigs, most of the plasma cells can be found in the crypts (Bianchi *et al.*, 1992; Stokes *et al.*, 1994) (figure 4).
A significant number of the immunoglobulin-producing plasma cells in the lamina propria secrete dimeric IgA antibodies that are linked to a J chain. The poly-immunoglobulin receptor, which is expressed on the basolateral membrane side of the epithelial cells binds the J chain covalently and is responsible for the transepithelial transport of dimeric IgA (as well as IgM which also contains a J chain) towards the luminal side. Once exposed onto the luminal side of the enterocytes, the poly-immunoglobulin receptor is cleaved and IgA, complexed to the cleaved part of the receptor (called secretory component) is released as secretory IgA into the lumen. This sIgA is protected from proteolysis by the secretory component and provides immune protection against pathogens (bacteria and viruses) by different mechanisms such as aggregation, neutralization and opsonization of pathogens and by blocking adhesion and toxins.
The most striking phenomenon of the mucosal immune system is the production of IgA by B cells. Although most B cells in the PP are membrane-IgM bearing B cells, the

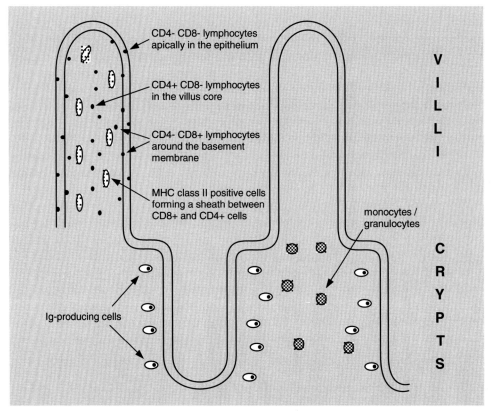

Figure 4. Schematic presentation of the small intestine with its distribution of lymphocytes in the lamina propria and the epithelium.

proportion of IgA⁺ B cells is here higher than in the peripheral lymph nodes. Experiments indicate that T cells as well as dendritic cells of the PP produce factors that induce switching of B cells upon antigenic stimulation preferentially from IgM to IgA. Cytokines such as IL-1, IL-5, IL-6 and TGF-β belong to these immunomodulating factors.

The caecal tonsils and the Meckel's diverticulum of the chicken
The chicken has only three organized lymphoid tissues along the gastrointestinal tract, namely the caecal tonsils, the Meckel's diverticulum and the bursa of Fabricius. The bursa of Fabricius is rather a pimary lymphoid organ and will not be discussed here. The caecal tonsil is localized in the luminal wall of the caeca at the ileo-caecal junction. It is the largest and most concentrated lymphoid tissue of the GALT and is like the PP organized into spherical units, each having a central crypt, diffuse lymphoid tissue and germinal centres (Schat and Myers 1991). The caecal tonsils are not present at hatching but develop, depending on the degree of antigenic stimulation, at the age of 2 weeks to reach their mature organization at the age of 5 to 7 weeks. Clustered and isolated T cells (35%) are found in the diffuse lymphoid tissue. B cells (45-55%) are

predominantly concentrated in B follicles (Sharma 1998). Although the number of B follicles is high, only few plasma cells are found in the caecal tonsils (Jeurissen *et al.*, 1994).

The Meckel's diverticulum is the remnant of the vitelline duct that extends between the yolk sac and the primitive gut of the embryo. Lymphoid infiltrates develop in the lamina propria of the remaining vitelline duct starting at the age of two weeks (Olah *et al.*, 1984). At all ages, the lumen of the Meckel's diverticulum remains connected to the small intestine by a small duct. Its general organization and function is very similar to that of the caecal tonsils (Jeurissen *et al.*, 1994).

The intestinal lamina propria of the chicken
Besides these organized lymphoid structures there exist in the chicken also aggregates of lymphocytes in the lamina propria. In the lamina propria, lymphocytes and macrophages are mostly concentrated in the loose connective tissue along the core of the villi, consisting of connective fibres, nerves, and blood and lymph vessels. Upon activation, this lymphoid tissue becomes organized as the caecal tonsils and the Meckel's diverticulum: the lymphocytes form distinct clusters of B cells and T cells and later on, germinal centres containing B cells (follicles), follicular dendritic cells and some T cells (Jeurissen *et al.*, 1994).

The intestinal epithelium
Another remarkable feature of the mucosal immune defence is the presence of IEL in the gut epithelium. They are morphologically separated form the underlying lamina propria lymphocytes by the basement membrane. In pigs, up to 27% of all epithelial cells have been shown to be IEL (T cells), 77% of which are $CD8^+$ and only 5% $CD4^+$ (Bianchi *et al.*, 1992; Stokes *et al.*, 1994). The $CD4^-/CD8^+$ T cells are mainly concentrated around the basement membrane while the $CD4^-/CD8^-$ T cells are positioned apically in the epithelium (Vega-Lopez *et al*, 1993) (figure 4). Moreover, 20% of freshly isolated IEL appear to be activated cells as evidenced by the expression of the α chain of the IL-2 receptor.

In the chicken 35% of the IEL are T cells, while 50% bear a B cell marker. However, no Ig-bearing cells were detected in the epithelium (Vervelde and Jeurissen, 1993). A remaining population (15%) of non-B, non-T, non-monocyte cells was present in all parts of the digestive tract. The total number of IEL increased up to 8 weeks after hatching and decreased thereafter. The number of IEL was highest in duodenum and jejunum, and decreased in the proximal part of the caecum and in the colon.

4.4. The acute-phase response: the induction of alarm signals

Inflammation is the answer of tissue to irritation, injury and infection. It consists of a complex cascade of non specific events, known as the acute-phase response, which confer early protection by limiting tissue injury to the place of infection or destruction: it controls the tissue injury, removes debris and initiates tissue restoration. One important function of this reaction is to recruit more phagocytic cells to the site of injury. Moreover, it initiates the specific immune response against the invader. The acute-phase response acts on a local as well as a systemic level.

4.4.1. The local response

The localized reaction is induced by clotting factors and pro-inflammatory cytokines released by the activated resident sentinels, the tissue macrophages. The combined actions of their pro-inflammatory cytokines IL-1, IL-6, IL-12 and TNF-α and the release of chemokines by activated macrophages and activated structural tissue cells (keratinocytes, fibroblasts, endothelial cells) are responsible for changes in the surrounding capillaries, inducing an influx of neutrophils, monocytes and effector lymphocytes into the site of inflammation. Indeed, there is an increase of specific adhesion molecules (E- and P-selectins) on the cell membrane of the endothelial cells, which trap the circulating leukocytes on the endothelium with subsequent diapedesis, and migration of these cells towards the place of tissue injury to fulfil their duty.

However, activated phagocytes release also other proteins with potent local effects, such as toxic radicals, peroxides, nitric oxide, plasminogen activator and phospholipase. Phospholipase A2 cleaves the fatty acid arachidonic acid (C20:4n6) from the glycerol backbone of membrane-bound phospholipids. The liberated arachidonic acid can then undergo controlled oxidative metabolism to form a variety of eicosanoids (C20) with different physiological and immune effects (figure 5). The cyclooxygenase pathway yields prostaglandins (PG), prostacyclin and thromboxanes while the lipoxygenase pathway the leukotrienes (LT) and lipoxins. The eicosanoids act as autocrine/paracrine regulators, since most of their biological effects are limited to the site of biosynthesis. LTB_4 stimulates chemotaxis of neutrophils and an increased expression of their C3b receptors while LTC_4, LTD_4 and LTE_4 are collectively known as the slow reactive substance of anaphylaxis (SRS-A), being more than 1000 times more potent than histamine in smooth muscle contraction and vasodilatation. The latter is important in view of the increased blood flow in inflamed tissues inducing an even higher influx of leukocytes into the inflammation site. After exerting their effect, eicosanoids are rapidly metabolised to inactive compounds in the liver and lungs.

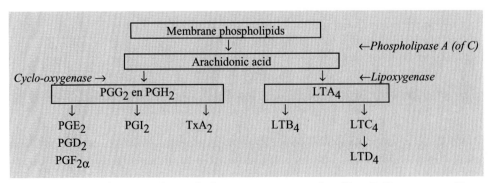

Figure 5. Arachidonic acid metabolism. PGE=prostaglandins, PGI=prostacyclins, TxA=thromboxanes, LT=leukotrienes.

4.4.2. The systemic response

The systemic part of the acute-phase response is induced by the pro-inflammatory cytokines IL-1, IL-6 and TNF-α, which have locally been released from the activated macrophages. They act on the hypothalamus inducing fever and loss of appetite, on the vascular endothelium releasing neutrophils from the bone marrow and the marginal pool into the blood, on fat and muscle mobilizing proteins and energy and on the liver inducing the release of acute-phase proteins in the blood plasma. Of the latter, C-reactive protein (CRP), serum amyloid A (SAA) and mannan-binding lectin are of particular interest as they opsonize bacteria and activate complement in a similar way as antibodies do.

4.5. Techniques for analysing intestinal health and immune activation

4.5.1. Epithelial cell turnover in the mucosal intestine

Determination of villus length and crypt depth
Tissue samples can be taken from mesenterial lymph nodes, spleen, ileum (with PP) and jejunum (with or without PP). Immediately after sampling, specimens are frozen by immersion in isopropanol-containing test tubes cooled in liquid nitrogen. Subsequently these samples are stored at -70°C until cryosections are made. Cryostat sections of 10μm thickness are picked up on slides, air-dried for 30 min, fixed in acetone for 5 min and stored at -70°C. Cryostat sections are stained directly or indirectly for expression of immunologically important molecules such as CD2, CD4, CD8, IgM, IgA, IgG, MHCII, Fc (antibody)-receptors, cytokines or others, with enzyme-, biotin or fluorochome-linked antibodies.
Tissue samples can also be fixed in phosphate buffered saline supplemented with 3.5% formaldehyde for 24 hours. The fixed specimens are then dehydrated by sequential submersions in ethanol baths (50%, 70%, 60%, 90%, 95%). Subsequently tissue blocks are incubated in a xylene and finally in paraffin. Paraffin-sections of 8 μm are rehydrated by following in reverse order, the previously described steps in ethanol baths.

Determination of apoptotic index
Apoptosis at the villus tops can be measured by identifying in situ, epithelial cells with fragmented DNA on tissue sections. Endonucleases generate free 3'-OH groups at the end of the fragmented DNA strands which can be detected by enzymatic labelling of the free 3'-OH termini with modified nucleotides (X-dUTP, X = biotin, digoxygenin or fluorescein). Suitable labelling enzymes include DNA polymerase and terminal deoxynucleotidyl transferase (TdT). Depending on the enzyme, these techniques are called respectively in situ nick translation (ISNT) and TdT-mediated X-dUTP nick end labelling (TUNEL). The fragmented DNA can then be visualised by labelled avidin,

anti-digoxygenin labelled antibodies or UV, depending on the X-dUTP used. The TUNEL method is currently applied on porcine intestinal specimens by Decuypere and Van Nevel (University of Ghent, Belgium).

Determination of mitotic index
In order to evaluate the turnover of the intestinal epihelium, mitotic indices of the cells of the crypts and villi can be determined in situ on tissue sections. The mitotic index is calculated on tissue sections of intestinal tissue by calculating the number of proliferating epithelial cells on the total number of epithelial cells. Therefore, the intestinal epithelium is analysed in situ on paraffin- or cryo-sections. In order to determine the proliferating cells in chickens (Krinke and Jamroz, 1996) and swine (Jin *et al.*, 1994) animals are given intravenously or intraperitoneally one hour before slaughter bromodeoxyuridine, a thymidine analog which is incorporated into newly synthesized DNA. The latter can then be visualized with labelled anti-bromodeoxyuridine antibodies. Proliferating intestinal cells can also be visualized by immunohistochemical staining for "proliferating cell nuclear antigen", Ki67, or thymidine kinase (Raab *et al.*, 1998; Preziosi *et al.*, 2000; Uni *et al.*, 1998a). The influence of non-digestible oligosaccharides on epithelial cell turn-over is for the moment under study by Decuypere and Van Nevel (University of Ghent, Belgium).

4.5.2. Detection of alterations in immune activity

The influence of specific nutrients or supplements can be analysed by defining immunological changes or responses in the mucosal (intestinal) or systemic immune system. These influences can be analysed on immune responses against specific antigens that have been intentionally administered during the trial period. Conversely, global changes in the immune status of the intestinal tract, such as cytokine activation, leukocyte (sub-) populations can also be measured.

Isolation of mononuclear cells from tissues (Van den Broeck et al., 1999)
For purifying mononuclear cells from porcine spleen and mesenterial lymph nodes, the respective organs are aseptically dissected and surrounding fat is removed. The mononuclear cells are isolated by teasing the tissue apart, followed by lysis of erythrocytes with ammonium chloride. The cells are pelleted and washed by repetitive centrifugation and resuspension and finally resuspended in leukocyte medium.
With respect to isolation of cells from the lamina propria of the pig the method is more elaborate. Segments of the small intestine are washed with calcium- and magnesium-free phosphate buffered saline (PBS) supplemented with EDTA to inhibit adherence of cells to matrix proteins. The segments are subsequently cut in small pieces and the cells are eluted from the tissues by an incubating treatment with collagenase. The isolated cells are then washed and resuspended as described above. For the isolation of mononuclear cells from PP, small intestine pieces are washed and incubated as done for the lamina propria. Cells are collected by scraping the PP and are subsequently washed and resuspended as described above.

Quantification of local cytokines
The influence of dietary products on the intestinal tract and in particular on its immune system can be analysed by determining changes in the local cytokine production. Cytokines can be quantified on the protein level or at the level of their transcription, namely mRNA. Quantifying cytokines in tissues at the protein level is however a difficult matter because of extraction and half-life. Procedures for their quantification at the mRNA level are easier.

In our laboratory in Ghent en Leuven, cytokines are quantified by on-line PCR on isolated cells from intestinal tissues or homogenates of the tissues themselves. Cells are isolated from intestinal tissues as described above. Total RNA is extracted with a commercial total isolation kit and mRNA is subsequently isolated on Qiagen columns. Total RNA and mRNA are quantified and purity examined by measuring optical densities at 260/280 nm. Reverse transcription to cDNA is accomplished with random hexamer primers. Quantitative on-line PCR is subsequently performed on the cDNA using sense/antisense primers specific for the targeted cytokines. A house-keeping gene such as cyclophiline is included as a quality control for the test sample cDNA. Besides the test samples, dilution series (number of copies/µl) of amplicons (plasmids containing the genes or specific fragments of the targeted cytokines, respectively) of the respective cytokines are amplified in order to produce for each cytokine a standard curve which enables the quantification of the cytokine (copy number) in the test samples. In order to define the specificity of the amplified product, melting temperature of each end product is determined at the end of each PCR reaction.

Quantification of local antigen-specific IgG, IgA and IgM-secreting cells: Elispot assay (Van den Broeck et al., 1999)
In this assay, antigen-specific antibody-secreting cells are enumerated in the cell suspensions from the tissues under study. For this purpose eluted cells are incubated in the wells of microtitre plates coated with the antigen in question. Each specific antibody-secreting cell can then deposit its antibodies on the surrounding antigen-coated plastic. After removing the cells, the antigen-bound IgA, IgM and IgG spots can be visualised after incubating the wells with their respective enzyme-labelled conjugates and addition of the substrate. In order to avoid diffusion of the converted substrate (colour), the last step is performed in low melting agar, so that coloured spots can easily be identified and counted.

Characterization and quantification of lymphocyte populations in isolated cells from tissue samples Mast et al., 1998a)
There exists a whole panel of monoclonal antibodies (MAb) for identifying respectively the different populations and subpopulations of chicken and porcine leukocytes. Alterations in their relative or absolute distribution in intestinal tissues and lymphoid organs under influence of dietary modulators can be examined in a fluorescence-activated flow cytometer. Isolated cells are first stained with their leukocyte (sub-)populations-specific MAb. After washing, cells are subsequently incubated with fluorochrome-labelled conjugates to identify the cell-bound MAb.

After a final wash, cells can be analysed for size, granularity and fluorescence (cell type) in the flow cytometer. For two colour analysis (analysis for two markers), MAb of different isotypes have to be selected which can subsequently be identified by their isotype-specific conjugates, labelled respectively with a different fluorochrome such as fluorescein, phycoerythrin or texas red.

In situ detection of lymphocyte (sub-)populations by immunohistochemistry (Mast et al., 1998a)
For single-colour in situ stainings, targeted antigens are demonstrated by using the relevant MAb and their respective labelled conjugates on cryostat sections.
For two-colour in situ stainings, cryostat sections are incubated for 45 min at room temperature with a mixture of the two relevant MAb defining respectively the target antigens. The MAb must be selected to belong to a different isotype. After washing, the sections are incubated with a mixture of an alkaline phosphate-labelled and a peroxidase-labelled conjugate, recognising respectively the different istopes of the primary antibodies. After washing, alkaline phosphatase activity is visualised first by incubating sections with its specific substrate and chromogen and peroxidase activity is developed thereafter by incubation with its specific substrate. Similar double staining results can be obtained by selecting primary antibodies that differ in species origin and using subsequently species-specific conjugates, or by using a directly and indirectly (with a conjugate) labelled antibody.

4.5.3. General systemic immune alterations: quantification of acute phase proteins in serum

The pro-inflammatory cytokines produced by activated macrophages induce indirectly a systemic immune alertness in the body. This immune alertness is accomplished by acute phase proteins produced by the liver on contact with pro-inflammatory cytokines, such as IL-1, IL-6 and TNF-α. Among the acute phase proteins CRP, haptoglobin and SAA are well known.
Commercial bioassays have been produced to measure these proteins. Haptoglobin can be quantified in a bioassay based on its interaction with methemoglobin or hemoglobin that results in peroxidase activity with the production of O_2 from H_2O_2. There exists also an ELISA test for haptoglobin that uses an anti-pig haptoglobin-specific antibody. CRP and SAA can be measured in commercial sandwhich ELISA's.

4.6. Induction of mucosal protection and modulation of immune responses towards the musosal surfaces

What kind of mucosal immune status is needed for optimal production and protection against pathogens, is not known. It is true that these two goals, production and protection, are quite often contradictory goals: indeed a high alerted immune status, even at mucosal surfaces, is quite often not beneficial for production as can be deduced from the chapter on the acute phase response. Induction and maintenance (continuous alertness) of protective immune mechanisms will always be at the cost of metabolic energy which is consequently lost for economic productive purposes. Nonetheless, a certain degree of mucosal immune alertness is needed to protect against chronic and acute infectious diseases that can cause major losses in production. Therefore in the next chapters we are analysing factors that can direct immune responses towards the mucosae or can improve a general mucosal alertness.

4.6.1. Dietary modulation of the eicosanoid biosynthesis

As we explained above (figure 5), arachidonic acid (C20:4n6) is liberated during the acute-phase response from membrane phospholipids by the action of phospholipase A2. The essential fatty acid (EFA) linoleic acid (C18:2n6) is the nutritional source for the generation of arachidonic acid containing phospholipids. Indeed, linoleic acid is converted by desaturases and elongases to eicosatetraenoic acid (C20:4n6) which is incorporated in membrane phospholipids. As linoleic acid is the predominant EFA in poultry feed, n-6 poly-unsaturated fatty acids (PUFA) are the primary products founds in tissue lipids. However when significant amounts of α-linolenic acid (C18:3n3) are fed to poultry, the concentration of n-3 PUFA increases with consequences in the composition of the membrane phospholipids. Nutritional intervention to modulate eicosanoid production is thus primarily mediated by competition of fatty acids for desaturases/elongases in PUFA formation, or by n-3 PUFA inhibition of cyclooxygenase (figures 6 and 7). Thus, the ratio of dietary n-3 to n-6 fatty acids determines the type and rate of eicosanoid production in leukocytes and accessory cells, and modulates the immune response. Feed ingredients high in n-6 PUFA include corn, vegetable oil and poultry fat while fish fat, fish meal and linseed oil are the major dietary source of n-3 fatty acids.

Fritsche et al., (1991) reported that feeding n-3 PUFA to growing leghorn chicks enhances the antibody response to sheep erythrocyte vaccinations but decreases mitogen-induced proliferation of lymphocytes. However, the same group found that broilers fed n-3 PUFA had reduced antibody-dependent cell-mediated cytotoxicity and tromboxane B formation in splenocytes compared to broilers fed n-6 PUFA (Fritsche and Cassity, 1992). It appears as if a decrease in the n-6/n-3 dietary PUFA ratio favors antibody responses over cell-mediated responses.

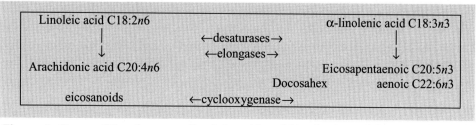

Figure 6. Competition between linoleic acid and linolenic acid for enzymes.

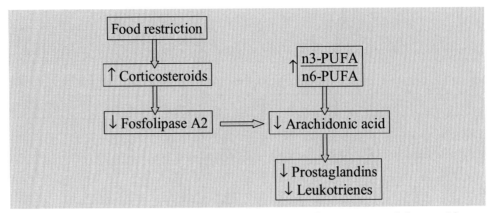

Figure 7. Influence of feed restriction and n3/n6 poly-unsaturated fatty acids on prostaglandin and leukotriene secretion.

Eicosanoids can be considered as regulators of macrophage activity and macrophage-lymphocyte interaction. Macrophages isolated from mice fed n-3 PUFA had lowered prostaglandin E_2 production and higher IL-1 and TNF-α when compared to macrophages fed n-6 PUFA (Lokesh et al., 1990). On the contrary, macrophages from broilers fed high levels of n-6 PUFA, released more IL-1 upon stimulation with *Staphylococcus aureus*, than macrophages from broilers fed diets high in n-3 PUFA (Korver and Klasing, 1997).

4.6.2. Influence of feed restriction on immune responsiveness

The immune system is part of the physiological system. They communicate with each other with the same molecules and with the same receptors and will thus influence each other. Although we are only beginning to study this intricate communication, neuroendocrine-immune interactions are already a hot topic in the mammalian (Blalock, 1994) and avian species (Marsh, 1992). Nutritional changes, shortages or absences (fasting) induce endocrine signals that will have an important impact on the immune system and responses.

Feed restriction and fasting is commonly practiced in the poultry industry for restricting growth and sexual maturity in breeders, for forcing moult in laying hens and for lowering heat-induced stress. Feed restricting or fasting induces increased levels of glucocorticoids, glucagon, insulin and growth hormone and decreased levels of thyroid hormones, having as a consequence a glucose decrease and free fatty acid increase in the blood. However, this endocrine alterations observed in chickens with feed restriction decrease with time suggesting that chickens quickly habituate to feed deprivation. Moreover, corticosteroid levels of fasted birds drop back to normal within 30 minutes following refeeding even if the refeeding period is as short as 5 seconds, or following only visual presentation of feed (Harvey and Klandorf, 1983).

But these increased corticosteroid levels have also an influence on the immune system. They are responsible for a detachment and redistribution of heterophils from the marginal pool (endothelium of the blood vessels) to the tissues (Gross and Siegel, 1986; Zulkifli et al., 1995). Moreover, glucocorticoids have an important impact on the transcription of cytokine and other genes that play an important role in immune responses. Indeed, the liposoluble glucocorticoids are able to pass through the cell membrane into cytoplasm of leukocytes where they can, after binding to their receptor, move towards the nucleus to associate with transcription-regulating sequences on DNA. The expression of as many as 1% of the genes might be regulated by glucocorticoids: they can either up-regulate or down-regulate the responsive genes. From an immunological point of view this is quite important as several cytokine genes are here the targets and can be down-regulated. Conversely, lipomodulin or lipocortin that suppresses phospholipase A2, is up-regulated with reduction of eicosanoids and resultant reduction in inflammatory responses.

Infection experiments with *Escherichia coli* and *Eimeria tenella* on chicks with ad libitum and restricted feeding (alternate day feeding) indicate that restricted feeding had beneficial effects on protection (survival) and weight gain (Katanbaf *et al.*, 1988; Ballay *et al.*, 1992, Zulkifli *et al.*, 1993). Similar restriction experiments demonstrated however no changes in specific antibody responses against sheep erythrocytes (Boa-Amponsem *et al.*, 1991). Conversely, Klasing (1988) observed an increase in anti-sheep erythrocyte antibodies in chicks that fasted 24 hours before or after antigen administration as compared to chicks fed ad libitum. Thus, it would appear that feed restriction has beneficial effects on protection against infections and that this is mediated by a reduction in arachidonic acid metabolites and most probably by modulation of some immune responses (figure 7).

4.6.3. Influence of some feed additives on immune responsiveness

Vitamin D and A

Vitamin D, its mode of action and its biological and immunological effects have extensively been reviewed by Van der Stede *et al.*, (2000a and b). Vitamin D is a complex of steroids that must undergo metabolic alterations to reach optimal biological activity. 25-hydroxyvitamin D_3 (25D3) appears to be the most active metabolite of vitamin D_3 that can be administered in feed for supporting cellular functions. Indeed, transport of vitamin D steroids after intestinal absorption is associated with vitamin D binding proteins that bind efficiently 25D3 but not the bio-active 1,25-dihydroxyvitamin D_3 (1,25D3). After passing through the cell and nuclear membranes, only bio-active vitamin D_3 can bind to the nuclear 1,25D3-receptor (VDR) and will exert its regulation of gene expression in target cells by binding to DNA D3-responsive elements (Soares *et al.*, 1995). The binding of VDR to its D3-responsive elements requires the presence of its ligand 1,25D3 and a companion protein, namely the RXR group of retinoic acid (vitamin A) receptors (figure 8) (DeLuca and Zierold, 1998). Although the active derivatives of vitamin A are not related to 1,25D3, their receptors VDR and RXR respectively, are members of the same superfamily of ligand-activated transcription factors (Carlberg and Saurat, 1996) and act together as heterodimers in their function. This demonstrates that vitamin D and vitamin A are linked in their signaling mechanisms. Indeed, it has been shown that the natural ligand for RXR, namely 9-cis

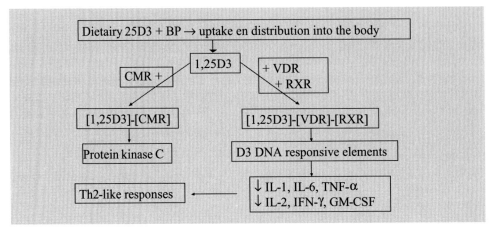

Figure 8. Mechamisms of Th2-like modulation by vitamine D3. CMR=cell membrane receptor, VDR=vitamine D3 receptor, RXR=retinoic acid receptor.

retinoic acid, suppresses both VDR-RXR binding to the DNA D3-responsive elements and 1,25D3-stimulated transcription (Haussler et al., 1995).

A unique membrane receptor for 1,25D3 has recently been detected on cell membranes (including intestinal epithelium cells) that mediates the rapid regulation of protein kinase C and does not appear to act via the traditional VDR (Nemere *et al.*, 1994, 1998). Moreover, *in vitro* experiments with chicken enterocytes have demonstrated an enhancement of tyrosine phosphorylation and rapid stimulation of mitogen-activated protein kinases by 1,25D3 and not 25D3 (de Boland and Norman, 1998). This unique membrane receptor might be important in view of the fact that 1,25D3 but not 25D3 reaches quickly toxic levels in feed.

Vitamin D is known for its anti-rachitic properties. Recently however, 1,25D3 has also been attributed with immunomodulatory capacities. Transplant rejection can be suppressed, and autoimmune diseases such as multiple sclerosis and rheumatoid arthritis can successfully be treated with vitamin D_3 and its analogs. They exert their effects on the immune system by regulating lymphocyte proliferation, differentiation of monocytes and secretion of cytokines as IL-2, granulocyte-macrophage colony-stimulating factor (GM-CSF) and INF-γ in T cells. As we have mentioned above, 1,25D3 modulates transcription of genes by binding with its receptor VDR to D3-responsive elements that can have enhancing or repressive effects on gene transcription. It inhibits production of macrophages-derived cytokines such as IL-1, IL-6 and TNF-α at the post-transcriptional level, most likely by reducing the half-life of specific mRNAs. The proliferation of T cells and the release of cytokines such as IL-2 and IFN-γ (Cippitelli and Santoni, 1998) are also suppressed by the reduced production of monocyte-derived T cell-activating cytokines (IL-1, TNF-α) and by direct action on the T cells. This is in agreement with experiments on pigs in our laboratory where simultaneous intramuscular injection of vitamin D_3 with an antigen enhanced the IgA and IgM responses in serum and the number of antigen-specific IgA and IgG antibody-secreting cells in the local draining lymph nodes (Van der Stede *et al.*, 2001).

Recently, the mechanism of GM-CSF repression has been elucidated and could be attributed to a two-hot process: firstly, VDR competes with NFAT1 (DNA-binding enhancer) for binding to the enhancer site, positioning itself adjacent to DNA-bound Jun-Fos (also a DNA-binding enhancer) and secondly by direct interaction with adjacent Jun-Fos on the DNA (Towers et al., 1999).

As we have already indicated above, vitamin A (retinol) might also influence the immune responsiveness and might even counteract the vitamin D action, as both vitamins interact directly or indirectly with RXR receptors. However, in vitro experiments in mice indicate that vitamin A inhibits secretion of Th1 cytokines (IFN-γ, GM-CSF, IL-2) but not Th2 cytokines (IL-4, IL-10), possibly through an inhibitory effect on protein kinase C activity (Frankenburg et al., 1998). This effect looks similar to vitamine D and opens also possibilities for modulating immune responses towards Th2 and consequently mucosae-directed immune responses such as IgA. This possibility has recently been confirmed in vivo whereby oral supplementation of vitamin A preserved mucosal IgA levels in protein-malnourished mice (Nikawa et al., 1999); retinoic acid restored the IL-5 level and the number of IL-4 and IL-5 containing cells in the small intestine which had been reduced by low-protein diet. Conversely, it has been demonstrated that vitamin A deficiency induces a Th1 priming environment with constitutive IL-12 and IFN-γ transcripts but devoid of constitutive IL-4 and IL-10 transcripts (Cantorna et al., 1995), and that this induction could be abolished by dietary retinoic acid supplementation. In conclusion, experimental data on vitamin A and D indicate a direction of the immune response towards Th2 that is known for activating antibody responses. Indeed immunization experiments in chickens and turkeys have indicated that dietary vitamin A supplementation up to levels of 6mg retinal equivalents per kg feed had beneficial effects on antigen-specific antibody responses (Sklan et al., 1994, 1995) whereas higher concentrations reduced the antigen-specific antibody responses. Moreover, studies in poultry indicate that severe vitamin A deficiency has a negative influence on intestinal functionality by reducing villus height and crypt depth and diminishing intestinal enzyme activities and that these negative effects could be restored by vitamin A repletion (Uni et al, 1998b, 2000).

β-glucans

In order to reduce or remove antibiotics and other prophylactic drugs in feed, there is a major search for immunomodulators (enhancers) that could be administered in feed. However, although some substances have promising potentials, the problem of passing undamaged the gastrointestinal tract and traversing the intestinal mucosa barrier remains a question. The mucosa-associated lymphoid tissue with its phagocytic M cells, seem to play here an important role especially for particles and macromolecules. One example of these immunomodulators is the group of β-glucans (table 3, figure 9) (reviewed by Vancaeneghem et al., 2000). Many studies in mammalians demonstrate that soluble and particulate β-glucans are immunological response modifiers and can be used in the therapy of experimental neoplasia, infectious diseases and immunosuppression. Their main direct target cells appear to be the monocyte/macrophage, neutrophil and natural killer cell. Glucan treatment of

Table 3. Important β-glucans, their origin and some general characteristics (Vancaeneghem *et al.* 2000).

Glucan	Origin	Mw (Da)	Helix	Solubility
	Fungus			
Krestin	*Coriolus versicolor*	1.10^5	Triple	?
Lentinan	*Lentinus edodus*	5.10^5	Triple	Gel
Schizophyllan	*Schizophillum commune*	$4,5.10^5$	Triple	Gel
Scleroglucan	*Sclerotium glucanum*	?	Triple	Soluble
Grifolan	*Grifola frondosa*	5.10^5	Triple + single	Gel
SSG	*Scerotinia sclerotionum*	$>2.10^6$	Triple	Soluble
	Glomerella cingulata	$6,8.10^5$	Triple	Soluble
	Yeast			
Macrogard	*Saccharomyces cerevisiae*	?	Non-uniform	Particle
Zymosan	*Saccharomyces cerevisiae*	?	?	Soluble
Betafectin (PPG)	*Saccharomyces cerevisiae*	?	?	Soluble
	Seaweed			
Laminarin	*Laminatia hypecborea*	?	Single	?
	Bacteriae			
Curdlan	*Alcaligenes faecalis*	?	?	Particle
	Algae			
	Euglena gracilis	5.10^5		?

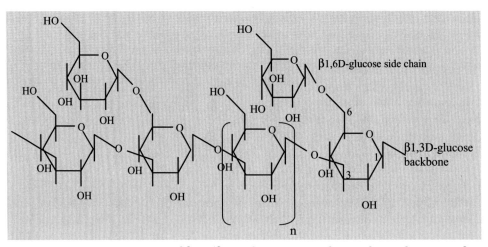

Figure 9. General structure of β1,3/β1,6-glucans. n is glucan-dependent: n=1 for SSG, n=2 for schizophyllan.

monocyte/macrophages induces the production of TNF-α, IL-1, platelet-activating factor and arachidonic acid metabolites, such as PGE_2 and LTB_4 (Abel and Czop, 1992; Doita *et al.*, 1991; Elstad *et al.*, 1994, Rasmussen *et al.*, 1990). The direct interaction of β-glucans with their target cells is mediated by cell membrane receptors, such as the lectin-binding domain of the (chain (CD11b) of the complement receptor 3 and the β-glucan receptors (Vetvicka *et al.*, 1996; Szabo *et al.*, 1995). Unfortunately, we have no knowledge of data on the influence of β-glucans on the avian immune system. Experiments in our laboratory in pigs with two different β-glucans have shown that their addition to the feed for two weeks after weaning reduced drastically the excretion of enterotoxigenic (F4[+]) *E. coli* (ETEC) upon ETEC challenge (figure 10) (Vancaeneghem S., Cox E. and Goddeeris B.M., unpublished data). Moreover, the effect of the two β-glucans on the immune system appeared completely different as evidenced by their different pattern of induction of cytokines (figure 11). Supplementation of glucans to the feed of piglets can also have a modulating adjuvant effect on simultaneously administered antigens. Also here had the different glucans different immunomodulating effects; one glucan shifted the systemic antibody response against an intramuscularly administered antigen towards IgA while the other suppressed the antigen-specific proliferation of peripheral blood leukocytes.

L-carnitine

Dietary L-carnitine (figure 12) supplementation was shown to exert an immunomodulatory effect on antigen-specific total Ig and IgG responses in growing chickens (Mast *et al.*, 2000; figure 13). The mechanism(s) accounting for the positive effect of L-carnitine on antibody production are currently not clear. Restoration of the cellular L-carnitine content might enhance the lipid metabolism and improve the

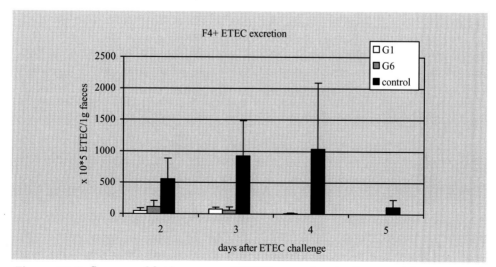

Figure 10. Influence of β-glucans on (ETEC) excretion in faeces. Piglets received glucan-containing feed for 2 weeks after weaning and were challenged 3 days later with ETEC.

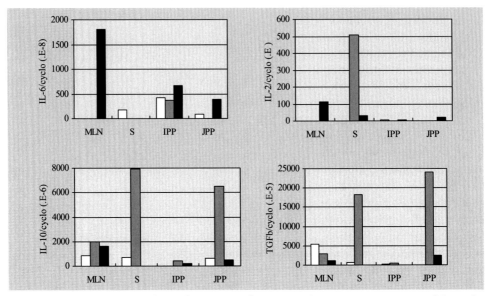

Figure 11. Cytokine profile of IL-6, TGFβ, IL-2 and IL-10 in mesenterial lymph node (MLN), spleen (S), ileal PP (IPP) and jejunal PP (JPP), 14 days after enterotoxigenic *E. coli* (ETEC) infection. Piglets received three different feeds (white bar = glucan 1; grey bar = glucan 6; black bar = no glucan) for 2 weeks after weaning and were challenged 3 days later with ETEC.

cellular energy balance. De Simone *et al.*, (1994) indicated that L-carnitine decreases the concentrations of cytokines, most notably TNF-α in man. In the rat models of cachexia and septic shock, L-carnitine treatment lowered IL-1β, IL-6 and TNF-α (Winter *et al.*, 1995). These cytokines play a pivotal role in general energy homeostasis, but also in the modulation of antibody responses. Finally, Di Marzio *et al.*, (1997) recently have shown that L-carnitine downregulates acidic sphingomyelase activity. This enzyme converts sphingomyelin into ceramide, an intracellular messenger molecule inducing apoptosis. Plausibly, L-carnitine also prevented apoptotic cell death of B and T lymphocytes during the immune responses of broiler chickens, which resulted in higher antibody titres

$$CH_3 - \overset{\overset{\displaystyle CH_3}{|}}{\underset{\underset{\displaystyle CH_3}{|}}{N^+}} - CH_2 - \overset{}{\underset{\underset{\displaystyle R}{|}}{CH}} - CH_2 - \overset{}{\underset{\underset{\displaystyle O^-}{|}}{C}}{=}O$$

Figure 12. Chemical structure of carnitine.

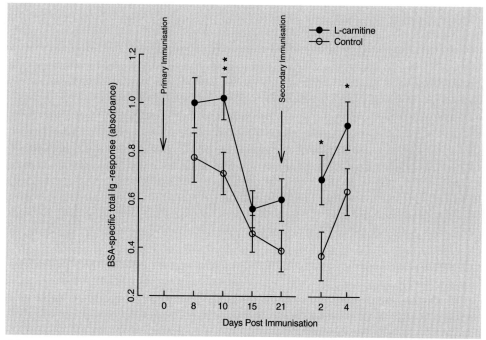

Figure 13. Influence of dietary L-carnitine supplementation on bovine serum albumine (BSA)-specific IgG responses. At each time point, mean absorbance with SEM was presented for n=28. The asterisk indicates a significant difference (P < 0.05) at 2 days post the secondary immunisation between mean IgG responses of broilers receiving an L-carnitine supplemented or a non-supplemented diet (control). (Mast *et al.*, 2000).

Dietary nucleotides
Until recently it was assumed that all living cells are capable to cover their requirements for nucleotides by de novo synthesis. Recent studies revealed however that in many tissues, except the liver, the requirement for nucleotides is covered not only by the de novo pathway but also by the salvage pathway that uses ribosyltransferases and kinases to add riboses and phosphates to already available nucleobases. The de novo synthesis of nucleotides is a time- and energy-consuming process. The uptake from the intestine of preformed nucleosides avoids the metabolic cost of the de novo biosynthesis. In the intestinal tract nucleotides can be partially absorbed in the gut. The greater proportion however is absorbed as nucleosides. In the gut cells, nucleosides are recombined with phosphoric acids to nucleotides and to nucleic acids. Partially the nucleosides and the nucleotides enter in the blood and are transported to different organs for the formation of new cells. Ribonucleic acids are also crucial in the synthesis of proteins and can be a limiting factor in the formation of proteins. Moreover, nucleotides play a major role in key functions of the organism, such as energy transport (ATP), enzyme function (e.g. coenzyme A) and intracellular messaging (cAMP or cGMP).

Investigations in laboratory animals and man have shown that the supplementation of nucleotides in the diet has major effects on the intestinal tract by accelerating growth and differentiation of the intestine, increasing the length of villi and improvement of the activity of brush border enzymes (Uauy *et al.*, 1990 and 1994). Moreover, dietary nucleotides seem to potentiate humoral as well as cellular immune responses (Jyonouchi *et al.*, 1993; Yamauchi *et al.*, 1996), resulting in increased resistance to pathogens (Kulkarni *et al.*, 1986). This effect is likely due to a requirement for preformed pyrimidines for proper development and activation of T cells (Kulkarni *et al.*, 1994). Experiments in mice have shown that dietary nucleotides may upregulate Th1 immune responses in systemic immunity as evidenced by decreased levels of serum IgE, IgG1/IgG2a ratio and splenic IL-4, a Th2 cytokine, and an increase in splenic IFN-γ, a Th1 cytokine (Nagafuchi *et al.*, 1997 and 2000). In addition studies demonstrated that infants fed a nucleotide-supplemented commercial formula developed a faecal flora with a predominance of bifidobacteria as opposed to enterobacteria with the unsupplemented formula (Uauy, 1994)

Experiments in swine have shown that supplementation of nucleotides in the feed (data on UNIMUN obtained from Dr. M. Verschaeve, Emma Nutrition, Belgium), gave better feed conversions, lower fat contents in carcasses and higher slaughter and "Carré" weights. Nucleotide supplementation in feed also decreased significantly mycotoxin levels in the liver. Moreover, pigs fed a nucleotide-supplemented feed have significant lower creatine kinase, lactate dehydrogenase and aspartate aminotransferase levels after stress than animals fed standard diet (data of Dr. M. Zomborsky, University of Kaposwar, Hungary, 1995).

4.6.4. *Protective and immunomodulatory effects of probiotics*

For livestock animals in the past improvement of production characteristics (growth and feed conversion) has been the main drive in selection of probiotics. In general, only minor contributions to increased 'performance' were gained especially for animals that were already kept in almost optimal conditions for growth and performance. However, presently not only performance is aimed at, but also other characteristics have gained in importance such as the ban on use of antimicrobial growth promoters in the EU, the increased emphasis on safety regulations for food production and an increased awareness for animal welfare and a sustainable agriculture, all of which have renewed the interest in more effective use of probiotics. As a consequence criteria now aim at management of microflora stability to prevent gastrointestinal tract disturbances, application with prefermented feed, and enhancement of colonisation resistance by competition for adherence, space and substrates with opportunistic and true pathogens.

The normal or indigenous flora of the intestines is in equilibrium with the physiology of the host animal. The intestinal microflora plays an important role in digestion of food and reduction of the risk of infections with specific pathogens (Dubos *et al.*, 1965). To facilitate the interactions between host and flora, the digested and undigested food serves as substrate for both. In addition, secretions such as mucus, saliva, gastric and pancreatic juices including a.o. enzymes, bile salts and secretory antibodies contribute to the interactions between all components of which many still are unidentified (Stewart *et al.*, 1993).

Role in the development of the immuun system and gut epithelium
The contribution of the microflora to the development of host elements such as the gut epithelia and the immune system is best illustrated in experimental settings where flora can be manipulated i.e. in germ free animals that lack any microflora element. The use of germ free and mono-contaminated animals has contributed largely to the understanding of the importance of the bacterial flora and bacterial antigens in the development of both the innate and the adaptive or specific immune system (Cebra, 1999; Umesaki *et al.*, 1999, Falk *et al.*, 1998). In germ free animals the development of especially the mucosal immune system and the gut is delayed as compared to either specific pathogen free (SPF) or conventional animals. Germ free animals that are exposed to the dangers of a conventional environment will attract diseases which have their main porte d'entrée via the mucosal surfaces and they generally will not survive this situation without severe precautions being taken. Even the young of SPF animals run a severe risk to attract fatal diseases in a conventional environment although they do have a selected gastrointestinal tract flora, which they received from the maternal animal. This indicates that a period of learning precedes the establishment of a stable host flora relationship to the benefit of both. Moreover, the microflora is pivotal in epithelial cell wall renewal, architecture, motility and differentiation of epithelial cells (Falk *et al.*, 1998). Mucosal epithelial cells can even be induced to produce specific lysins (Lopes-Boada *et al.*, 2000). The gut ecosystem created in this way may be the answer to the complex mechanism of colonisation resistance and competitive exclusion.

The flora is contained within a lumen of which the gut wall cell populations exhibit a high rate of turnover. As a consequence, adhesion of flora components is a transient phenomenon. After renewal of the gut wall, recruitment of the flora components from the lumen is required to maintain a cell wall related flora. The high rate of turnover simultaneously decreases the opportunities for infectious agents and pathogens to invade the body. Gut motility is also important for throughput and removes all unwanted and unabsorbed material. The gut flora influences gut motility as has been shown in experiments with germ free and conventional animals. It appeared that entero-endocrine effects that are related to the composition of the flora lead to differences in responsiveness of the neuromuscular complex that in germ free animals can be reversed by addition of a conventional flora. In this way the presence of a microbial flora leads to limitation of the exposure time to pathogens present in the gastrointestinal tract (Huseby *et al.*, 1994; Strandberg *et al.*, 1996).

Interaction between the gut flora and mucosa: cytokine induction
Carbohydrate binding proteins both on mammalian cells and on bacteria provide active mutual interaction sites. The species-specific glycosylation of mucosal lining plays a role in sensitivity to pathogens and in selection of indigenous flora elements (Kelly and King, 1991; King, 1995). Lectins are widespread in feed and food (recently reviewed by Woodley, 2000). Lectins of plant or bacterial origin are proteins that can

bind to poly- and oligosaccharides and to sugar moieties that are present on glycosylated proteins of any kind. In that way they compete with carbohydrate binding sites for beneficial and for potentially pathogenic bacteria and for toxins present in the gut. In this way lectins present in the food or feed may alter the microbial ecology of the gut. Probiotic micro-organisms may interfere or compete with these interactions in a host beneficial way (Falk *et al.*, 1998). Toll receptors, first recognised in embryogenesis, are membrane proteins important for recognition of innate defence mechanisms by binding of e.g. lipopolysaccharides and lipoteichoic acids. The recognition by toll-like receptors in general leads to induction of inflammatory responses mediated by cytokines such as IL-1. Such receptors are present on antigen-presenting cells (macrophages) but also on gut epithelial cells (Cario *et al.*, 2000). It is envisaged that this is one of the pathways to generate so called danger signals by epithelial cells. Unknown receptor interactions in which specific receptors and ligands may be involved may lead also to induction of IL-8 (chemokine) in epithelial cells. The release of this chemokine leads to the recruitment of cells from the innate and specific immune system to the location of interaction (Steiner *et al.*, 2000). Probiotics that enhance or promote induction of such cytokines might be beneficial to the host as it offers a pre-emptive strike. For *Lactobacillus* strains and other non-pathogenic bacteria this has been demonstrated in vivo and in vitro by Maassen *et al.* (1999, 2000) and Haller *et al.* (2000). The primary function of such inflammatory cytokines is recruitment of leukocytes but in addition some cytokines like TNF-β may also have a direct interaction with pathogens (killing).

Anaerobic flora components as probiotics
The effect of the chloroform-resistant intestinal microflora (CRM) on the intestines and immune system in other species than the mouse has yet not been investigated in much detail. Preliminary studies in gnotobiotic pigs clearly indicate that the effect of the CRM component of the intestinal microflora is similar in pigs as its counterpart is in mice (J. Sinkora, personal communication). The CRM is composed of spore-forming anaerobic bacterial species, mainly *Clostridia* and segmented filamentous bacteria (SFB) (Umesaki *et al.*, 1999). At this moment the CRM component that is best characterised are the SFB. In all genera of the animal kingdom including chicken (Yamauchi and Snel, 2000), pigs (Sandford, 1991) and cattle (Smith, 1997), SFB have been shown (Klaasen *et al.*, 1993a). The SFB are mainly localised on the epithelia, which cover the Peyer's patches in mice and rats (Klaasen *et al.*, 1992). SFB promote phenotypic differentiation of IEL and enhance the number of IgA$^+$ plasma cells in the mucosa of the small intestine (Moreau *et al.*, 1982; Klaasen *et al.*, 1993b; Talham *et al.*, 1999). In addition, SFB enhanced the concanavalin A-induced proliferation of mesenteric lymph node cells (Klaasen *et al.*, 1993b). Also the presence of cultivable *Clostridia* promotes an enhancement of the number of IgA$^+$ plasma cells and IEL. Recently, SFB were also found to give a strong stimulus to the transit of intestinal contents through the small intestine (Snel *et al.*, 1996). Moreover, increased mitotic activity as well as an increase in the ratio of the number of columnar epithelial cells to the number of goblet cells in the small intestine can be shown. It has been concluded that SFB are important indigenous bacteria for the development of the

mucosal architecture (Umesaki *et al.*, 1995). The important contribution of CRM and SFB therein to host beneficial health effects may lead to investigation of their potential use under those conditions in husbandry where natural transfer may be hampered by unfavourable environmental conditions such as in SPF or high hygiene standard pig husbandry.

Probotics in the chicken and the pig
In the chicken, most interest has gone to the exclusion of micro-organisms that are pathogenic to the human consumer rather than to poultry (*Salmonella, Campylobacter*). Tolerance to a certain level and resistance to infection is observed for these pathogens. The role of the flora therein was demonstrated in that the flora of infection-resistant adult birds was able to confer this resistance to young animals (Impey and Mead, 1989). Similarly, effects of a partial protective flora were observed with other micro-organisms such as *Campylobacter jejunum* and *Clostridium spp*. It was thought that the resistance was mediated by competitive exclusion to which many different micro-organisms contributed (Mead and Impey, 1986). From the complex mixtures no specific competitors have been isolated. A similar approach as for *Salmonella* has been tried for *E. coli* with similar results. Investigations in our laboratory (W.J.A. Boersma and M.E. Koenen) were initiated on the in vitro selection of immuno-enhancing probiotic bacteria for application in the chicken. To this end enhancement by selected lactobacilli of an a-specific (mitogen concanavalin A) activation of spleen lymphocytes was used (figure 14). It could be demonstrated that the *Lactobacillus*

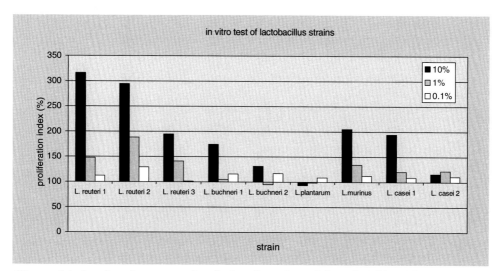

Figure 14. In vitro immunostimulation by selected lactobacilli. Spleen cells of layer chickens were sub-optimally stimulated with concanavalin A. The cells were co-cultured or not with three concentrations of lactobacilli of test strains. The cells were labelled during 4h incubation with ^{3}H thymidine. A stimulation index expressed as a percentage was calculated that corrected for incorporation of ^{3}H thymidine by lactobacilli alone.

strains selected in vitro, also had an immuno-enhancing effect in vivo when the humoral response to a model antigen was evaluated (figure 15).

At birth, the pig gut is characterised by a lack of immunological cell types characteristic of the mature gut. The gnotobiotic pig shows a similarly immature architecture (Rothkoetter and Pabst, 1989). These cellular subsets appear at clearly defined time points and in an ordered sequence (Vega-Lopez et al., 1995, Joling et al., 1994). It has been assumed that the CRM microflora includes bacteria that are highly important for animal health. It also has been shown that these bacteria are extremely sensitive to antibiotics (Klaassen et al., 1992). Therefore, it has been suggested that the application of antibiotics included as feed additives may result in a disturbed intestinal physiology and a suboptimal development of the immune system, due to its adverse effect on CRM populations in the piglet. The slow immunological maturation of the gut in the young may provide a partial explanation for the negative environmental effects experienced during this period. These negative aspects are further compounded by management practices in intensive husbandry (weaning at a relatively early age, transport, mixing, unstable ranking). Early weaning in particular has been implicated as a period prone to intestinal disturbances. It has been reported that early weaning is associated with reduced immunological function of the peripheral as well as the mucosal immune system in piglets, including changes in the composition of T cells

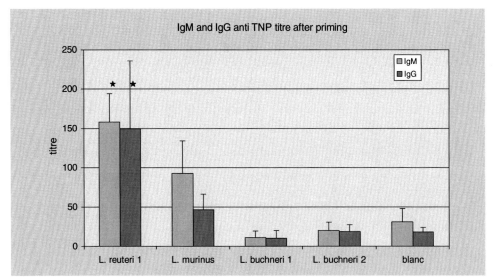

Figure 15. In vivo immuno-stimulation of systemic humoral immune responses of layer chicken by selected lactobacilli. Lactobacilli were orally administered during five consecutive days (10^9/day). The chickens were subsequently immunised with a sub-optimal dose of trinitrophenylised keyhole limpet hemocyanin (KLH-TNP). IgG and IgM anti-TNP titres were determined in serum at several time-points (indicated day 7). The chickens fed with L. reuteri had a significant higher response than was observed in chickens fed with buffer only (blank)

in the lamina propria (Bailey *et al.*, 1992). As a consequence of these negative factors experienced in a particularly vulnerable stage of life, health risks such as infection increase. This results in decreased animal welfare and production. The luminal content has a major influence on the functioning of the gut. Parenteral feeding in humans leads to gut atrophy, changes in morphology and increase in the frequency of T-lymphocytes, an indication for increased danger signals along the gastrointestinal tract (Matzinger, 1998). Weaning-associated inflammatory processes along the gut show increased level of IL-1 and fibrinogen (Cummins *et al.*, 1988). Similar phenomena were also observed in post-weaning piglets (McCracken *et al.*, 1995). In addition increased numbers of CD4[+] T-helper cells were found (Pluske *et al.*, 1999). Such changes were accompanied by typical morphological changes in the gut (McCracken *et al.*, 1999).

For pigs the immunological aspect of probiotics have been investigated only to a limited extend. Most studies on probiotics are directed to intervention strategies that aim to attain competitive exclusion for specific pathogens (reviewed by Mulder *et al.*, 1997). Though it cannot be excluded that immunological mechanisms play a role therein, thus far that has not been investigated in any detail. In our laboratory (W.J.A. Boersma and M.E. Koenen) a similar stategy as was pursued in chicken, is followed for the selection of immuno-enhancing probiotics for pigs.

4.7. References

Abel, G. and J.K. Czop, 1992. Stimulation of human monocyte β-glucan receptors by glucan particles induces production of TNF-alpha and IL-1. International Journal of Immunopharmacology 14, 1363-1373.

Bailey, M., C.J. Clarke, A.D. Wilson, N.A. Williams, C.R. Stokes, 1992. Depressed potential for interleukin-2 production following early weaning of piglets. Veterinary Immunology and Immunopathology 34, 197-207.

Ballay, M., E.A. Dunnington, W.B. Gross and P.B. Siegel, 1992. Restricted feeding and broiler performance: age at initiation and length of restriction. Poultry Science 71, 440-447.

Bianchi, A.T.J., R.J. Zwart, S.H.M. Jeurissen and H.W.M. Moonen-Leusen, 1992. Development of the B- and T-cell compartments in porcine lymphoid organs from birth to adult life: an immunohistochemical approach. Veterinary Immunology and Immunopathology 33, 201-221.

Binns, R.M. and R. Pabst, 1988. In: Husband, A.J. (Editor), Homing and migration of lymphoid cells. CRC Press, FL, vol.2, p.137.

Binns, R.M. and R. Pabst, 1994. Lymphoid tissue structure and lymphocyte trafficking in the pig. Veterinary Immunology and Immunopathology 43, 79-87.

Binns, R.M. and S.T. Licence, 1985. Patterns of migration of labelled blood lymphocyte populations: evidence for two types of Peyer's patches in the young pig. Advances in Experimental Medicine and Biology 168, 661-668.

Blalock, J.E., 1994. The syntax of immune-neuroendocrine communication. Immunology Today 15, 504-511.

Boa-Amponsem, K., N.P. O'Sullivan, E.A. Gross, E.A. Dunnington and P.B. Siegel, 1991. Genotype, feeding regimen, and diet interactions in meat chickens. 3. General fitness. Poultry Science 70, 697-701.

Cantorna, M.T., F.E. Nashold, and C.E. Hayes, 1995. Vitamin A deficiency results in a priming environment conductive for Th1 cell development. European Journal of Immunology 25, 1673-1679.

Cario, E., I.M. Rosenberg, S.L. Brandwein, P.L. Beck, H.C. Reinecker and D.K. Podolsky, 2000. Lipopolysaccharide activates distinct signaling pathways in intestinal epithelial cell lines expressing toll-like receptors. Journal of Immunology 164, 966-772.

Carlberg, C. and J.H. Saurat, 1996. . Vitamin D-retinoid association: molecular basis and clinical applications. Journal of Investigative Dermatology. Symposium Proceedings 1, 82-86.

Cebra, J.J., 1999. Influences of microbiota on intestinal immune system development. American Journal of Clinical Nutrution 69, 1064S-1051S

Chang, C.F. and P.B. Hamilton, 1979. The thrombocyte as the primary circulating phagocyte in chickens. Journal of the Reticuloendothelial Society 25, 585-590.

Cippitelli, M. and A. Santoni, 1998. Vitamin D3: a transcriptional modulator of the interferon-gamma gene. European Journal of Immunology 28, 3017-3030.

Cummins, A.G., T.W. Steele, J.T. Lbrooy and D.J.C. Shearman, 1988. Maturation of the rat small intestine at weaning. Changes in the epithelial cell kinetics, bacterial flora and mucosal immune activity. Gut 29, 1672-1679.

de Boland, A.R. and A.W. Norman, 1998. $1\alpha,24(OH)2$-vitamin D3 signaling in chick enterocytes: enhancement of tyrosine phosphorylation and rapid stimulation of mitogen-activated protein (MAP) kinase. Journal of Cellular Biochemistry 69, 470-482.

De Simone, C., G. Famularo, S. Tzantzoglou, V. Trinchieri, S. Moretti, and F. Sorice, 1994. Carnitine depletion in peripheral blood mononuclear cells from patients with AIDS: effect of oral L-carnitine. AIDS 8, 655-660.

DeLuca, H.F. and C. Zierold, 1998. Mechanisms and functions of vitamin D. Nutrition Reviews 56, S4-10, S54-75.

Di Marzio, L., E. Alesse, P. Roncaioli, P. Muzi, S. Moretti, S. Marcellini, G. Amicosante, C. De Simone, and M.G. Cifone, 1997. Influence of L-carnitine on CD95 cross-lining-induced apoptosis and ceramide generation in human cell lines: correlation with its effects on purified acidic and neutral sphingomyelinases in vitro. Proceedings of the Association of American Physicians 109, 154-163.

Doita, M., L.T. Rasmussen, R. Seljelid and P.E. Lipsky, 1991. Effect of soluble aminated β-1,3-D-polyglucose on human monocytes: stimulation of cytokine and prostaglandin E2 production but not antigen-presenting function. Journal of Leukocyte Biology 49, 342-351.

Dubos, R., W.R. Schaedler, R. Costello, P. Hoet, 1965. Indigenous, normal and autochtonous flora of the gastrointestinal tract. Journal of Experimental Medicine 122, 59-66.

Elstad, M.R., C.J. Parker, F.S. Cowley, L.A. Wilcox, T.M. McIntyre, S.M. Prescott and G.A., Zimmerman, 1994. CD11b/CD18 integrin and a β-glucan receptor act in concert to induce the synthesis of platelet-activating factor by monocytes. Journal of Immunology 152, 220-230.

Falk, P.G., L.V. Hooper, T. Midvedt and J.I. Gordon, 1998. Creating and maintaining the gastrointestinal ecosystem: what we know and need to know from gnotobiology. Microbiology and Molecular Biology Reviews 2, 1157-1170.

Frankenburg, S., X. Wang, and Y. Milner, 1998. Vitamin A inhibits cytokines produced by type 1 lymphocytes in vitro. Cellular Immunology 185, 75-81.

Fritsche, K.L. and N.A. Cassity, 1992. Dietary n-3 fatty acids reduce antibody-dependent cell cytotoxicity and alter eicosanoid release by chicken immune cells. Poultry Science 71,1646-1657.

Fritsche, K.L., N.A. Cassity, and S. Huang, 1991. Effect of dietary fat source on antibody production and lymphocyte proliferation in chickens. Poultry Science 70, 611-617.

Gross, W.B. and P.B. Siegel, 1986. Effect of initial and secondary periods of fasting on heterophil/lymphocyte ratios and body weight. Avian Diseases 30, 345-346.

Haller, D, C. Bode, W.P. Hammes, A.M. Pfeifer, E.J. Schiffrin and S. Blum, 2000. Non-pathogenic bacteria elicit a differential cytokine response by intestinal epithelial cell/leucocyte co-cultures Gut 47, 79-87.

Harvey, S. and H. Klandorf, 1983. Reduced adrenocortical function and increased thyroid function in fasted and refed chickens. Journal of Endocrinology 98, 129-135

Haussler, M.R., P.W. Jurutka, J.C. Hsieh, P.D. Thompson, S.H. Selznick, C.A. Haussler and G.K. Whitfield, 1995. New understanding of the molecular mechanism of receptor-mediated genomic actions of vitamin D hormone. Bone 17, 33s-38s.

Huseby, E., P.M. Hellstrom and T. Midvedt, 1994. Intestinal microflora stimulates myoelectric activity of rat intestinal wall by promoting cyclic initiation and aboral propagation of migrating myoelectric complexes. Digestive Diseases and Sciences 39, 946-956.

Impey, C.S. and G.C. Mead, 1989. Fate of salmonellas in the alimentary tract of chicks pre-treated with a mature caecal microflora to increase colonization resistance. Journal of Applied Bacteriology 66, 469-75

Jeurissen, S.H.M., L. Vervelde and E.M. Janse, 1994. Structure and function of lymphoid tissues of the chicken. Poultry Science Reviews 5, 183-207.

Jin, L., L. P. Reynolds, D.A. Redmer, J.S. Caton, J. D. Crenshaw, 1994. Effects of dietary fiber on intestinal growth, cell proliferation, and morphology in growing pigs. Journal of Animal Science 72, 2270-2278.

Joling, P, A.T.J. Bianchi, A.L. Kappe, and R.J. Zwart, 1994. Distribution of lymphocyte subpopulations in thymus, spleen, and peripheral blood of specific pathogen free pigs from 1 to 40 weeks of age. Veterinary Immunology and Immunopathology 40, 105-117.

Jyonouchi, H, L. Zhang-Shanbhag, M. Georgieff and Y Tomita, 1993. Immunomodulating actions of nucleotides: enhancement of immunoglobulin production by human cord blood lymphocytes. Pediatric Research 34, 565-571.

Katanbaf, M.N., D.E. Jones, E.A. Dunnington, W.B. Gross, and P.B. Siegel, 1988. Anatomical and physiological responses of early and late feathering broiler chickens responses to various feeding regimes. Archiv für Geflugelkunde 68, 344-351.

Kelly, D. and T.P. King, 1991. The influence of lactation products on the temporal expression of histo-blood group antigens in the intestine of suckling pig: lectin histochemical and immunohistochemical analysis. Histochemical Journal 23, 55-60.

King, T.P., 1995. Lectin cytochemistry and intestinal epithelial cell biology. In: A. Pusztai and S Bardocz (editors), Lectins: Biomedical Perspective. Taylor & Francis. London, U.K., pp.183-210.

Klaasen, H.L., J.P. Koopman, M.E. Van den Brink, M.H. Bakker, F.G. Poelma, and A.C. Beynen,. 1993a. Intestinal, segmented, filamentous bacteria in a wide range of vertebrate species. Laboratory Animals 27, 141-50.

Klaasen, H.L., P.J. Van der Heijden, W. Stok, F.G. Poelma, J.P. Koopman, M.E. Van den Brink, M.H. Bakker, W.M. Eling, and A.C. Beynen, 1993b. Apathogenic intestinal segmented filamentous bacteria stimulate the mucosal immune system of mice. Infection and Immunity 61, 303-306.

Klaasen, H.L., J.P. Koopman, F.G. Poelma, A.C. Beynen, 1992. Intestinal segmented filamentous bacteria. FEMS Microbiological Reviews 8, 165-180.

Klasing, K.C., 1988. Influence of acute feed deprivation or excess feed intake on immunocompetence of broiler chicks. Poultry Science, 67, 626-634

Korver, D.R. and K.C. Klasing 1997. Dietary fish oils alters specific and inflammatory immune responses in chicks. Journal of Nutrition 127, 2039-2046.

Krinke, A.L. and D. Jamroz, 1996. Effects of feed antibiotic Avoparcine on organ morphology in broiler chickens. Poultry Science 75, 705-710.

Kulkarni, A.D., F.B. Rudolph and C.T. Vanburen, 1994. The role of dietary sources of nucleotides in immune function - A review. Journal of Nutrition 124, S1442-S1446.

Kulkarni, AD, W.C. Fanslow, F.B. Rudolph and C.T. Van Buren CT, 1986. Effect of dietary nucleotides on response to bacterial infections. Journal of Parenteral and Enteral Nutrition 10, 169-171.

Lokesh, B.R., T.J. Sayers, and J.E. Kinsella, 1990. Interleukin-1 and tumor necrosis factor synthesis by mouse peritoneal macrophages is enhanced by dietary n-3 polyunsaturated fatty acids. Immunology Letters 23, 281-285.

Lopez-Boada, Y.S., C.L. Wilson, L.Hooper, J.I. Gordon, S.J. Hultgren and W.C. Parks, 2000. Bacterial exposure induces and inactivates matrilysin in mucosal epithelial cells. Journal of Cell Biology 148, 1305-1315.

Maassen, C.B.M., J.D. Laman, M.J. Heijne den Bak-Glashouwer, F.J. Tielen., J.C.P.A. van Holten-Neelen, L. Hoogteijling, C. Antonissen, R.J. Leer., P.H. Pouwels, W.J.A. Boersma, and D.M. Shaw, 1999. Instruments for oral disease-intervention strategies: recombinant lactobacillus casei expressing tetanus toxin fragment C for vaccination or myelin proteins for oral tolerance induction in multiple sclerosis. Vaccine 17, 2117-2128.

Maassen, C.B.M., J.D. Laman, W.J.A. Boersma, and Claassen E., 2000 Modulation of cytokine expression by lactobacilli and its possible therapeutic use. In: R. Fuller and G. Perdigon (editors), Probiotics 3, Immunomodulation by the gut microflora and probiotics. Kluwer. London, pp. 176-193.

MacDonald, T.T. and P.B. Carter, 1982. Isolation and functional characteristics of adherent phagocytic cells from mouse Peyer's patches. Immunology 45, 769-774.

Marsh, J.A., 1992. Neuro-endocrine interactions in the avian species - A review. Poultry Science Reviews 4, 129-167.

Mast, J. and B.M. Goddeeris B.M., 1999. Development of immunocompetence of broiler chickens. Veterinary Immunolology and Immunopathology 70, 245-256.

Mast, J. and B.M. Goddeeris, 1998a. CD57, a marker for B-cell activation and splenic ellipsoid-associated cells of the chicken. Cell and Tissue Research 291, 107-115.

Mast, J. and B.M. Goddeeris, 1998b. Immunohistochemical analysis of the development of the structural organisation of chicken spleen. Vlaams Diergeneeskundig Tijdschrift 67, 36-44.

Mast, J., J. Buyse and B.M. Goddeeris, 2000. Dietary L-carnitine supplementation increases antigen-specific immunoglobulin (Ig) G in broiler chickens. British Journal of Nutrition 83, 161-166.

Matzinger, P., 1998. An innate sense of danger. Seminars in Immunology 10, 399-415.

McCracken, B.A., M.E. Spurlock, M.A. Roos, F.A. Zuckermann and R.H. Gaskins 1999. Weaning anorexia may contribute to local inflammation in the piglet small intestine. Journal of Nutrition 129, 6136-619.

McCracken, B.A., R.H. Gaskins, P.J. Ruwe-Kaiser, K.C. Klasing and D.E. Jewell, 1995. Diet dependent and diet independent metabolic responses underlie growth stasis of pigs at weaning. Journal of Nutrition 125, 2838-2845.

Mead, G.C. and C.S. Impey, 1986. Current progress in reducing salmonella colonization of poultry by competitive exclusion. Society for Applied Bacteriology symposium series 15, 67S-75S.

Moreau, M.C., P. Raibaud and C. Muller, 1982. Relation entre developpement du systeme immunitaire intestinal a IgA et l'etablissement de la flora microbienne dans le tube digestif du souriceau holoxenique. Annales d'Immunologie (Pasteur) 133D, 29-39.

Mulder, R.W.A.W., R. Havenaar and J. Huis in 't Veld, 1997. Intervention strategies: the use of probiotics and competitive exclusion microflora's against contamination with pathogens in pigs and poultry. In: R. Fuller (editor), Probiotics 2. Applications and practical aspects. Chapman & Hall, London, U.K., pp.186-207.

Nagafuchi, S., M. Totsuka, S. Hachimura, M. Goto, T. Takahashi, T. Yajima, T. Kuwata and S. Kaminogawa, 2000. Dietary nucleotides increase the proportion of a TCR gamma delta (+) subset of intraepithelial lymphocytes (IEL) and IL-7 production by intestinal epithelial cells (IEC); Implications for modification of cellular and molecular cross-talk between IEL and IEC by dietary nucleotides. Bioscience Biotechnology and Biochemistry 64, 1459-1465.

Nagafuchi, S., T. Katayanagi, E. Nakagawa, T. Takahashi, T. Yajima, A. Yonekubo and T. Kuwata, 1997. Effects of dietary nucleotides on serum antibody and splenic cytokine production in mice. Nutrition Research 17, 1163-1174.

Nemere, I, M.C. Dormanen, M.W. Hammond, W.H. Okamura, and A.W. Norman, 1994. Identification of a specific binding protein for 1(,25-dihydroxyvitamin D3 in basel-lateral membranes of chick intestinal epithelium and relationship to transcaltachia. Journal of Biological Chemistry 269, 23750-23756.

Nemere, I., Z. Schwartz, H. Pedrozo, V.L. Sylvia, D.D. Dean and B.D. Boyan, 1998. Identification of a membrane receptor for 1,25-dihydroxyvitamin D3 which mediates rapid activation of protein kinase C. Journal of Bone and Mineral Research 13, 1353-1359.

Nikawa, T., K. Odahara, H Koizumi, Y. Kido, S. Teshima, K. Rokutan and K. Kishi, 1999. Vitamin A prevents the decline in immunoglobulin A and Th2 cytokine levels in small intestine mucosa of protein-malnourished mice. Journal of Nutrition 129, 934-941.

Olah, I, B. Glick and R.L. Taylor, 1984. Meckel's diverticulum. II. A novel lymphoepithelial organ in the chicken. The Anatomical Record 208, 253-263

Pabst, R. and R.M. Binns 1989. Heterogeneity of lymphocyte homing physiology: several mechanisms operate in the control of migration to lymphoid and non-lymphoid organs in vivo. Immunological Reviews 108, 83-109.

Pabst, R., M. Geist, H.J. Rothkötter and F.J. Fritz, 1988. Postnatal development and lymphocyte production of jejunal and ileal Peyer's patches in normal and gnotobiotic pigs. Immunology 64, 539-544.

Pluske, J.R., R.H. Gaskins, P.C.H. Morel, D.K. Revell, M.R. King and E.A.J. James, 1999. The number of villus and crypt CD4+ cells in the jejunum of piglets increases after weaning. In: P.D. Cranwell (editor), Manipulating Pig Production VII, p.244. Australian Pig Science Association, Werribee, Australia

Preziosi, R., G. Sarli and P.S. Marcato, 2000. Cell proliferation and apoptosis in the pathogenesis of oesophagogastric lesions in pigs. Research in Veterinary Science 68,189-196.

Raab, S., R. Leiser, H. Kemmer, R. Claus, 1998. Effects of energy and purines in the diet on proliferation, differentiation, and apoptosis in the small intestine of the pig. Metabolism 47, 1105-1111.

Rasmussen, L.-T., J. Fandrem and R. Seljelid, 1990. Dynamics of blood components and peritoneal fluid during treatment of murine E. coli sepsis with β-1,3-D-polyglucose derivatives. Scandinavian Journal of Immunology 32, 330-340.

Rothkötter, H.J. and R. Pabst, 1989: Lymphocyte subsets in jejunal and ileal Peyer's patches of normal and gnotobiotic minipigs Immunology 67, 103-108. Immunology. 67, 103-108

Sanford, S.E., 1991. Light and electron microscopic observations of a segmented filamentous bacterium attached to the mucosa of the terminal ileum of pigs. Journal of Veterinary Diagnostic Investigations 3, 328-333.

Schat, K.A. and T.J. Myers, 1991. Avian intestinal immunity. Critical Reviews in Poultry Biology 3, 19-34.

Sharma, J.M., 1998. Avian immunology. In: Pastoret P.P., P. Griebel, H. Bazin and A. Govaerts (editors), Handbook of vertebrate immunology. Academic Press, London, pp. 73-136.

Sklan, D., D. Melamed and A. Friedman, 1994. The effect of varying levels of dietary vitamin A on immune response in the chick. Poultry Science 73, 843-847.

Sklan, D., D. Melamed and A. Friedman, 1995. The effect of varying dietary concentrations of vitamin A on immune response in the turkey. British Poultry Science 36, 385-392.

Smith, M.W. and M.A. Peacock, 1992. Microvillus growth and M-cell formation in mouse Peyer's patch follicle-associated epithelial tissue. Experimental Physiology 77, 389-392.

Smith, TM, 1997. Segmented filamentous bacteria in het bovine small intestine. Journal of Comparative Pathology 117, 185-190.

Snel, J., M.E. Van den Brink, M.H. Bakker, F.G.J. Poelma and P.J. Heidt, 1996. The influence of indigenous flora on small intestinal transit time in mice. Microbiology and Ecology in Health and Disease. 9, 207-214

Soares, J.H. Jr, J.M. Kerr and R.W. Gray, 1995. 25-hydroxycholecalciferol in poultry nutrition. Poultry Science 74, 1919-1934.

Steiner, T.S., J.P. Nataro, C.E. Poteet-Smith, J.A. Smith and R.L. Guerrant, 2000. Enteroaggregative E.coli expresses a novel flagellin that causes IL-8 release from intestinal epithelial cells. Journal of Clinical Investigations 105, 1769-1777.

Stewart, C., K. Hillman, F. Maxwell, D. Kelly and T.P. King, 1993. Recent advances in probiosis in pigs: observations on the microbiology of the pig gut. In: Garnsworthy and D.J.A. Cole (editors), Recent advances in animal nutrition. Nottingham University Press, Nottingham, U.K., pp. 197-219.

Stokes, C.R., M. Bailey and A.D. Wilson, 1994. Immunology of the porcine gastrointestinal tract. Veterinary Immunology and Immunopathology 43, 143-150.

Strandberg, K., G. Sedvall, T. Midvedt, and B.E. Gustafsson, 1966. Effect of soem biologically active amines on the cecum wall of germ free rats. Proceedings of the Society for Experimental Biology and Medicine 121, 699-702.

Szabo, T., J.L. Kadish and J.P. Czop, 1995. Biochemical properties of the ligand-binding 20-kDa subunit of the β-glucan receptors on human mononuclear phagocytes. Journal of Biological Chemistry 270, 2145-2151.

Talham, G.L., H.Q. Jiang, N.A. Bos and J.J. Cebra 1999. Segmetned filamentous bacteria are potent stimuli of a physiologically normal state of the murine gut mucosal immune system. Infection and Immunity 67, 1992-2000

Towers, T.L., T.P. Staeva and L.P. Freedman, 1999. A two-hit mechanism for vitamin D3-mediated transcriptional repression of the granulocyte-macrophage colony-stimulating factor gene: vitamin D receptor competes for DNA binding with NFAT1 and stabilized c-Jun. Molecular and Cellular Biology 19, 4191-4199.

Uauy, R., 1994. Nonimmune system responses to dietary nucleotides. Journal of Nutrition 124, S157-S159.

Uauy, R., G. Stringel, R. Thomas and R. Quan, 1990. Effect of dietary nucleosides on growth and maturation of the developing gut in the rat. Journal of Pediatric Gastroenterology and Nutrition 10, 497-503.

Uauy, R., R. Quan and A. Gil, 1994. Role of nucleotides in intestinal development and repair - Implications for infant nutrition. Journal of Nutrition 124, S1436-S1441.

Umesaki, Y., H. Setoyama., S. Matsumoto, A. Imaoka and K. Itok, 1999. Differential roles of segmented filamentous bacteria and clostridia in development of the intestinal immune system. Infection and Immunity 67, 3504-3511.

Umesaki, Y., Y. Okada, S. Matsumoto, A. Imaoka and H. Setoyama, 1995. Segmented filimentous bacteria are indigenous intestinal bacteria that activate intraepithelial lymphocytes and induce MHC class II molecules and fucosyl asialo GM1 glycolipids on the small epithelial cells in the ex-germfree mouse. Microbiology and Immunology 39, 555-562.

Uni, Z., R. Platin and D. Sklan, 1998a. Cell proliferation in chicken intestinal epithelium occurs both in the crypt and along the villus. Journal of Comparative Physiology B 168, 241-247.

Uni, Z., G. Zaiger and R. Reifen, 1998b. Vitamin A deficiency induces morphometric changes and decreased functionality in chicken small intestine. British Journal of Nutrition 80, 401-407.

Uni, Z., G. Zaiger, O. Gal-Garber, M. Pines, I. Rozenboim and R. Reifen, 2000. Vitamin A deficiency interferes with proliferation and maturation of cells in the chicken small intestine. British Poultry Science 41, 410-415.

Van den Broeck, W., E. Cox and B.M. Goddeeris, 1999. Induction of immune responses in pigs following oral administration of purified F4 fimbriae. Vaccine 17, 2020-2029.

Van der Stede, Y., E. Cox and B. Goddeeris, 2000a. 1,25 dihydroxyvitamine D3. Deel 1: structuur, werking en biologische effecten. Vlaams Diergeneeskundig Tijdschrift 69, 218-228.

Van der Stede, Y., E. Cox and B. Goddeeris, 2000b. 1,25 dihydroxyvitamine D3. Deel 2: rol in het immuunsysteem. Vlaams Diergeneeskundig Tijdschrift 69, 229-233.

Van der Stede, Y., E. Cox, W. Van den Broeck and B.M. Goddeeris, 2001. Enhanced induction of IgA in pigs by calcitriol after intramuscular immunisation. Vaccine 19, 1870-1878.

Vancaeneghem, S., E. Cox, P. Deprez, S. Arnouts and B.M. Goddeeris, 2000. β-glucanen als immunostimulantia en als adjuvantia. Vlaams Diergeneeskundig Tijdschrift 69, 412-421.

Vega-López, M.A., E. Telemo, M. Bailey, K. Stevens and C.R. Stokes, 1993. Immune cell distribution in the small intestine of the pig: immunohistochemical evidence for an organized compartmentalization in the lamina propria. Veterinary Immunology and Immunopathology 37, 49-60.

Vega-Lopez, M.A., M. Bailey; E. Telemo and C.R. Stokes, 1995. Effect of early weaning on the development of immune cells in the pig small intestine. Veterinary Immunology and Immunopathology 44, 319-327.

Vervelde, L. and S.H.M. Jeurissen, 1993. Postnatal development of intra-epithelial leukocytes in the chicken digestive tract: phenotypical characterisation in situ. Cell and Tissue Research 274, 295-301.

Vetvicka, V., B.P. Thornton and G.D. Ross, 1996. Soluble β-glucan polysaccharide binding to the lectin site of neutrophil or natural killer cell complement receptor type 3 (CD11b/CD18) generates a primed state of the receptor capable of mediating cytotoxicity of iC3b-opsonized target cells. Journal of Clinical Investigations 98, 50-61.

Winter, B.K., G. Fiskum and L.L. Gallo, 1995. . Effects of L-carnitine on serum triglyceride and cytokine levels in rat models of cachexia and septic shock. British Journal of Cancer 72, 1173-1179.

Woodley, J.F., 2000. Lectins for gastrointestinal targeting -15 years on. Journal of Drug Targeting 7, 325-333

Yamauchi, K.E. and J. Snel, 2000. Transmission electronmicroscopic demonstration of phagocytosis and intracellular processing of segmented filamentous bateria by intestinal epithelial cells of the chick. Infection and Immunity 68, 6496-6504.

Zulkifli, I., E.A. Dunnington, W.B. Gross, A.S. Larsen, A. Martin and P.B. Siegel, 1993. Responses of dwarf and normal chickens to feed restriction, Eimeria tenella infection and sheep red blood cell antigen. Poultry Science 72, 1630-1640.

Zulkifli, I., H.S. Siegel, M.M. Mashaly, E.A. Dunnington and P.B. Siegel, 1995. Inhibition of adrenal steroidogenesis, neonatal feed restriction and pituitary-adrenal axis response to subsequent fasting in chickens. General and Comparative Endocrinology 97, 49-56.

5. Nutritional management to prevent disorders in post-weaning pig health

H.M.G. van Beers-Schreurs[1] and E.M.A.M. Bruininx[2]
[1] *Department of Farm Animal Health, Pig Health Unit, Utrecht University, PO Box 80.151 3508 TD Utrecht*
[2] *Research Institute for Animal Husbandry, PO Box 2176 8204 AD Lelystad*

Introduction

Despite a considerable amount of research in the past, post-weaning problems such as the well known growth depression and the occurrence of diarrhoea and nervous signs, often followed by death, are still wide spread in modern pig husbandry. Some of the post weaning problems are due to presence of specific infectious agents like Streptococcus species, however most of the post-weaning problems may be part of the Post Weaning syndrome (PWS), which include post-weaning diarrhoea (PWD), oedema disease (OD), and endotoxin shock. Vellenga (1989) estimated the extra annually costs of PWS within the Dutch pig husbandry to be about 11 million Euros. Today these yearly costs are estimated to be about 7 million Euros due to improvements in housing conditions, management, nutrition, and the use of anti microbial growth promoters (AMGP). However, the costs of the PWS syndrome may again increase due to a more critical use of anti microbial growth promoting agents at present and a possible ban in the future. Therefore, further research is warranted on factors that maintain the health of the weaned pig.

The aim of this paper is to review the mechanisms by which feed and feeding strategy improves the health status of the gastro-intestinal tract of the pig. After a short introduction about health problems of weanling piglets the process of weaning will be described in chapter 2. Research models available to study different aspects of gastro-intestinal health are described in chapter 3. In chapter 4 and 5 the nutritional management and suggestions for formulation of the diet will be discussed. Practical considerations of water and feed are described in chapter 6 and the conclusions are given in chapter 7.

5.1. Health problems of weanling piglets

In just weaned piglets multiplication of pathogenic *Escherichia coli* may result in diarrhoea, in piglets with nervous signs (OD) or in sudden death as reviewed earlier (Van Beers-Schreurs et al 1992). Nervous signs such as incoordination, tremor, paralysis, and paddling can also be seen in piglets suffering from meningitis caused by *Streptococcus suis* (Windsor 1977). The symptoms of these diseases will be more pronounced by the presence of other infectious agents like Rotaviruses. These agents damage the epithelial layer of the intestine and cause diarrhoea (Bohl et al. 1979, Tzipori et al 1980).

5.1.1. Pathogenesis of health problems of weanling piglets

Various agents may threat the health status of the weanling piglet. Most of these agents, and more specific, the bacterial and protozoan agents are known for their permanent presence on the pig farm. Multiple predisposing factors determine whether an infectious agent displays its infective properties or not. Other agents, for example influenza viruses, enter the swineherd and cause a lot of health disorders, like coughing, fever, and less appetite (Brown et al 1992). In general, after a few weeks most of the pigs will develop antibodies and show no clinical signs anymore.

The most important agents in the weanling period are *E. coli* and *S. suis*. It is known that these agents are considered to be endemic in the swineherd and therefore the young piglet will contact these agents early in life. During the foetal period the gastro-intestinal tract (GIT) of the pig is sterile. Searching for milk, the pig contacts sow's faeces, the contaminated vulva and other parts of the sow. A few hours after birth the GIT will be contaminated and colonisation of the GIT starts. The pigs' immunity determines whether the potential pathogenic agents will reach the GIT and whether they are able to enter the body by passage of the mucosal barriers of the intestinal wall. In general the immune system can be divided in an a-specific and a specific part. For the GIT, the a-specific immune system consists of a well-developed barrier system and the specific immune system relies on specific antibodies against pathogenic agents.

5.1.2. Barriers of the gastro-intestinal tract

Infectious agents may enter the body by several pathways. The oral-nasal system is widely accepted as 'porte d'entrée'. Beside this route, the agents may enter the body through the umbilical cord or lesions caused by fighting or by human intervention e.g. cutting off the tail or teeth. The agents that attack the GIT enter the body by oral uptake. From the moment of uptake till passing the body with the faeces the potential pathogen has to cope with a lot of barriers: the stomach, the motility of the small intestine, the mucosal defence in the small intestine and the resistance to colonisation in the large intestine. In the stomach the pH is very low, and at low values, most bacteria (not viruses) will be inactivated. Passing the stomach, the bacteria enter the duodenum, where the pH is neutralised by bicarbonate from the pancreas. In order to become pathogenic the agent has to find a place in the small intestine to colonise. However, the motility in the small intestine and therefore the passage time of the digesta is most of the time so high that colonisation cannot take place. Moreover, in order to reach the enterocytes, the bacteria have to resist the natural mucosal defence (Lecce et al, 1982). The so-called 'glycocalyx' has to be penetrated. This glycocalyx consists mainly of sialic acid-containing glycoproteins. The chemical nature of the mucins and number of goblet cells depend on the presence of offending substrates (Brown et al, 1988). In good health, mucosal surfaces are constantly bathed by secretions loaded with antibacterial enzymes and antibodies, which impede the attempts of pathogens to colonise the surface (Beachey, 1981). In this layer the carbohydrate portion provides receptors for the E. coli. The bounded bacteria will be mixed up with the chyme in the intestine. Bacteria that enter the large intestine are able to colonise because the passing time of the bacteria in the large intestine is higher and there is a surplus of fermentable digesta. Whether specific bacteria are able to colonise or not also depends on the composition of the diet and on the competition between bacteria. As long as the flora in the large intestine is stable, it is almost impossible for potentially pathogenic bacteria to multiply in the large intestine. This is what is called: resistance to colonisation (Van der Waaij et al 1971, Bouvee-Oudenhoven et al. 1997)

5.1.3. The immune system of the young pig

Since the specific immune system of the young pig is anatomically and functionally immature, survival is dependent on the passive transfer of maternal antibodies by colostrum and milk (Stokes and Bourne, 1989). Thus newborn pigs are especially vulnerable to pathogenic challenge during the period in which antibody levels have declined in milk before the active immune mechanisms are developed. Since Immunoglobulin G (IgG) constitutes the major immunoglobulin in serum, the predominant immunoglobulin isotype in colostrum is IgG. As colostrum secretion ends and lactation proceeds, IgG decreases quickly and IgA becomes the major immuoglobulin isotype in sow milk (Stokes and Bourne, 1989). IgA is produced in the mammary gland and is resistant to intestinal degradation. IgA provides protection by neutralising viruses and inhibiting bacterial attachment (Porter, 1986). However, during lactation the pig is only protected against those antigens that the sow has previously developed immunity to. The active immunity in the piglets' intestine does not develop until 4 - 7 weeks of age (Gaskins and Kelley, 1995).

5.2. The process of weaning and its influence on the health status

At weaning the pigs will be separated from the sow, mixed and housed in another pen. This, together with the change of diet (no milk supply anymore), is a situation the pig can hardly handle. Due to the change in diet, the piglet stops receiving antibodies from the sow and the a-specific barrier is weakened by several mechanisms.
In order to keep the pH of the stomach as low as possible, the feed intake of the pig should be regular. However, change of diet may result in a period of fasting (as described later), followed by a period of 'over-eating'. During the latter period the stomach will be filled and emptied too fast to keep the pH at a low level. Subsequently, bacteria will pass the stomach and enter the small intestine.
The small intestine looses its integrity in the first few days after weaning. Microscopic examination shows shortened villi with the minimum height at day four after weaning

and increased crypt depth at eleven days after weaning (Cera et al, 1988a, Van Beers-Schreurs et al 1998b). The latter is expected to be the result of the shortening of the villi just after weaning (Nabuurs 1993). The crypt cells have to proliferate at a higher rate to restore the shortened villi. Several investigators have been searching for the cause of the villus atrophy. In the early eighties it was suggested that the reduction in the numbers of enterocytes could be the result of an increased rate of cell loss. The physical effects of the diet (as will be discussed later) or the changes in blood supply to the villi could cause additional losses of senescent apical villus enterocytes (Tasman-Jones et al 1982). However, experiments with gnotobiotic piglets have shown that the stunted villi observed after diet changes are the result of a decreased production of new cells in the crypts and not of an accelerated loss of mature enterocytes from the surface of the villi due to a villus-damaging mechanism (Hall and Byrne 1989). Rotaviruses may cause villus atrophy. Viral replication occurs primarily in villus enterocytes, resulting in hyper-regenerative villus atrophy (Bohl, 1979). More recently it became clear that feed intake in particular is an important factor. McCracken et al. (1995), Van Beers-Schreurs (1998a) and Pluske (1996a, b) showed the interdependence between voluntary feed intake and mucosal architecture. In Table 1 the effect of post weaning energy intake level on villus height (expressed as the percentage of villus height at weaning), as reported in literature is shown.

Providing milk at the level of energy intake resulting from the ad libitum provision of a dry diet resulted in similar villus atrophy. However, when piglets were given free

Table 1. The relative effect of early post weaning energy intake on average villus height in the small intestine of pigs (Bruininx et al., 2001a).

Author	Energy source	Energy intake	Age at weaning	Age at slaughter	Villus height (weaning = 100%)
Pluske et al., 1996a	starter diet	5.7 MJ GE[†]/d	28 d	33 d	- 30%
Pluske et al., 1996a	ewes' milk	7.4 MJ GE/d	28 d	33 d	- 2%
Pluske et al., 1996b	cows' milk	2.3 MJ GE/d	29 d	34 d	- 27%
Pluske et al., 1996b	starter diet	5.1 MJ GE/d	29 d	34 d	- 18%
Pluske et al., 1996b	cows' milk	5.2 MJ GE/d	29 d	34 d	- 4%
Pluske et al., 1996b	cows' milk	8.9 MJ/GE/d	29 d	34 d	+ 11%
Pluske et al., 1996c	cows' milk	5.5 MJ/GE/d	28 d	33 d	- 4.8%
Kelly et al., 1991	starter diet	2.9 MJ GE/d	14 d	20 d	- 55%
Van Beers, 1998a	starter diet	0.53 MJ ME[‡]/BW$^{0.75}$/d	28 d	32 d	- 40%
Van Beers, 1998a	sows' milk	0.48 MJ ME/BW$^{0.75}$/d	28 d	32 d	- 35%
Van Beers, 1998a	sows' milk	1.4 MJ ME/BW$^{0.75}$/d	28 d	32 d	- 11%

[†] GE = Gross energy

[‡] ME = Metabolizable energy

access to cow's milk (2.5 times maintenance) or sow's milk ad libitum, pre- and post-weaning villus heights were similar (Pluske, 1996b, Van Beers-Schreurs et al, 1998a). This suggests that when feed/energy intake is maintained after weaning, the typical villus atrophy at 4 to 5 days after weaning can be avoided.

The shortening of the villi does not only affect the absorptive capacity of the small intestine, but also the digestive capacity. The villus atrophy coincides with a loss of enzyme activity (Hampson, 1986, Smith, 1984). Furthermore, it has been shown that digestive enzymes are present in insufficient quantities and quality for the changes in dietary composition that occur (Lindemann *et al.*, 1986; Makkink, 1993). Thus, the changes in the intestinal morphology and function are associated with post weaning maldigestion and malabsorption (Kenworthy, 1976, Hampson and Kidder, 1986, Nabuurs, 1993).

Maldigestion and malabsorption result in accumulation of fluid and digesta in the small intestine. The osmotic activity of the digesta increases and the absorption of water will further decrease. Due to a larger volume, the small intestines are extended, resulting in an increased motility of the intestinal wall. Subsequently, the digesta has less time to be digested. The overflow of undigested and unabsorbed nutrients reach the colonic area and there they 1) will be fermented by microbial agents, 2) may act as substrate for pathogenic strains of E. coli *and* 3) will enhance the osmotic activity, possibly resulting in osmotic diarrhoea (Alpers 1992).

In piglets suffering from diarrhoea in the first week post weaning, pathogenic E. coli strains have passed the stomach and have colonised the small intestine. However, colonisation of the small intestinal tract by E. coli strains coming from lower down the intestinal tract has also been described (Hampson, 1985). The pathogenic strains of E. coli colonise the intestinal wall by adherence. This adherence is a prerequisite for infectivity (Beachey, 1981). A number of fimbrial adhesins have been described, of which F4 is the best known. F4-positive enterotoxigenic E. coli strains can produce plasmid-coded heat-labile (LT) enterotoxins (Smith and Hall, 1967). LT increases the cyclic AMP concentration and probably causes diarrhoea by both inhibiting absorption and stimulating secretion, using cyclic AMP as intracellular messenger (Field, 1981). This gives rise to a net secretion of water, sodium, chloride and bicarbonate ions. Another enterotoxin, the heat -stable toxin increases the production of cyclic guanosine monophosphate, leading to secretion of water and electrolytes.

In piglets suffering from nervous signs these signs may be caused by OD caused by endotoxins or meningitis caused by S. suis. Proliferation of E. coli and probably S. suis in the large intestine occurs due to the malabsorption and maldigestion of nutrients as described earlier. What is known of the pathogenesis of OD is that it is associated with enterotoxinaemic strains of E. coli and with the occurrence of vascular degeneration and oedema in several organs. The reason why the symptoms of OD and Streptococci meningitis are apparent in the second week after weaning, whereas PWD is seen in the first week after weaning has been unclear for years. It is suggested that the permeability of the mucosal barrier is higher at approximately ten days after weaning; under normal circumstances it is impossible for large amounts of endotoxins to pass the mucosal barrier. Recently, scientist of ID Lelystad have confirmed that the permeability of the small intestinal wall on days 10-14 after weaning is higher than on other days after weaning (Niewold et al, 2000). These authors suggest that the higher permeability is caused by a reduction in cardiovascular capacity and thus the cardiovascular adaptability (Niewold et al, 2000). The modern pig seems to be unable to deal with a reduction in blood-flow, due to the redistribution of blood-flow as happens in stressed pigs. The lower cardiac output and stress may lead to anoxia in the epithelium of the intestinal wall. Oxidative phosphorylation is blocked and anaerobic glycolysis results in lactic acid production, acidaemia, and intracellular acidosis (Schumer and Erve, 1975). This together with an increased demand of oxygen at two weeks after weaning may result in ischaemia and in increasing intestinal permeability (as discussed by Niewold et al 2000). The increased permeability enhances translocation of toxins produced by Escherichia *coli* strains (Berg 1992) and probably enhances the translocation of S. *suis*. The toxins of E. *coli* damage vascular cells and post mortem examination shows oedema of the submucosa of the cardial gland region of the stomach, eyelids, mesocolon, full stomach as well as arteriopathy and focal encephalopathy (Terpstra, 1958, Timoney, 1950, Nielsen, 1986, Svendsen, 1974). The predominant lesions caused by S. *suis* are neutrophilic meningitis or encephalitis and suppurative bronchopneumonia (Higgins and Gottschalk, 1999). Although the pathogenesis of these diseases is not exactly the same, they have the onset of the pathogenesis in common: the process of weaning.

In order to prevent health problems in weaned piglets the circumstances at weaning have to been improved. This can be achieved be improving the housing and hygienic conditions and facilitate an easy change of diet at weaning.

5.3. Research models to study several aspects of gastro-intestinal integrity

In general gastro-intestinal integrity is dependent on villus-crypt ratios and the permeability of the intestinal wall. Lot of research work is done to measure these parameters at the time of weaning

5.3.1. Villus-crypt ratio's

As shown in table 1 several authors measured villus height and crypt depth of intestinal tissue at various days after weaning. The method of sampling is described earlier by Nabuurs (1993). This ratio or the absolute heights and depths could be considered as a result of what have could happened before sampling. However, the method of sampling implicates killing of piglets as long as we are not capable of sampling the jejunum of unanesthetized animals that have not been surgically treated before. The disadvantages of this kind of study (cross sectional) could be overcome by a longitudinal study, in which the same animals are sampled every three or for days. Unfortunately, these methods are not available.

5.3.2. Absorptive capacity/Permeability of the gastro-intestinal wall

The absorptive capacity of the gastro-intestinal wall of un-anaesthetized pigs can be measured by adding small inert molecules (markers) to the diet. The amount of marker leaving the body by the non-rectal route could be considered as absorbed. Catheterization of for example the portal vein and sampling blood for analysis of short-chain acids (SCFA) proved to be a valid method to measure the absorption of these SCFA (Rerat 1985). However, catheterisation of pigs takes place under anaesthesia and the influence of the anaesthesia and the surgical treatment itself could have influenced the integrity of the intestinal tract.

Parsons has already described principles of in vivo methods for investigation of intestinal absorption in 1968. The fistula method, by which absorption can be measured in the undisturbed, conscious trained pig by introducing known amounts of material into the fistula and measuring the quantity recovered after a suitable time. In 1946 Sols started experiments in which infusion of segments was involved. In 1994 Nabuurs described a modification of the experimental work of Solz and developed the Small Intestine Segment perfusion test (SISP) for measuring net absorption along the intestinal tract at various sites.

In vitro methods to measure permeability of tissue have been developed fifty years ago. Nowadays the method developed by Ussing (1951) known as Ussing Chambers is still very popular. In principle this method consists of reducing the electrochemical potential gradient across the epithelial layers to zero by exposing the two faces of the tissue to identical bathing solutions and clamping the transcellular potential difference at a value of zero volts.

5.4. Nutritional management of the pre- and post weaning pig

5.4.1. Early post weaning feed intake

It is generally accepted that weaning is a stressful event (e.g. Worsaae and Schmidt, 1980). At weaning, piglets are removed from the dam and reallocated to another pen. After weaning, the piglets are provided with solid feed in a way that is completely different from suckling milk. As mentioned earlier, the piglet may respond to weaning by refraining from eating (Bark et al., 1986). Le Dividich and Herpin (1994) recognised a period of underfeeding immediately after weaning. They concluded that the metabolizable energy requirement for maintenance (MEm) was not met until day 5 post-weaning. These findings were confirmed by Bruininx (unpublished data; Figure 1). Using feeding stations for weanling piglets Bruininx showed that an average metabolizable energy intake of 461 $kJ.kg^{-0.75}.d^{-1}$ was attained at d 6 after weaning.

Apart from the low energy intake during the first days post weaning, Van Diemen et al. (1995), Gentry et al. (1997), Moon et al. (1997) and Sijben et al. (1997) showed a tendency to an increase in energy requirements for maintenance during the first week after weaning. Averaged over these studies the MEm requirement was 461 $kJ.kg^{-0.75}.d^{-1}$

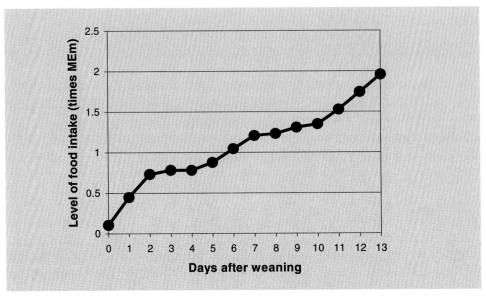

Figure 1. Interval between weaning and the day on which weanling piglets meet the MEm requirement of 461 kJ.kg$^{-0.75}$.d^{-1} (Bruininx,unpublished data).

during week 1 post weaning and 418 kJ.kg$^{-0.75}$.d^{-1} averaged over the subsequent five weeks.

In addition to the variation in feed intake observed among groups of weanling piglets, Brooks (1999) showed a great variation in feed intake traits within groups. Even though the majority of pigs had started eating within five hours after weaning some pigs took a very long time (up to 54 h) before they started eating. These findings were confirmed by Bruininx et al. (2001b) using feeding stations to monitor individual feed intake of group housed weanling piglets. These authors found that within 4 hours after weaning, approximately 50% of the pigs started eating, whereas it lasted about 50 hours before 95% of all pigs had started eating.

Therefore, it can be concluded that during the first days after weaning piglets strongly depend on body energy reserves due to the low energy intake. Moreover, the energy requirements during the first week post weaning are elevated due to a reallocation of energy towards maintenance. Apart from the low feed intake, a large variation in feed intake among individual animals seems to be present. In the following paragraphs of this chapter the nutritional management of the pre- and post weaning pig will be discussed. As mentioned earlier, early post weaning feed intake is considered to be an important factor in the pathogenesis of the PWS that is associated with villus atrophy. Therefore, the next sections will focus on (pre- and post weaning) factors that may stimulate (early) feed intake by the weaned pig.

5.4.2. Pre-weaning feed intake

To ease the transition from milk during the sucking period to a solid diet after weaning, piglets frequently are given feed while they are still nursing (= creep feeding). Although several authors assessed the strategy of creep feeding (Hampson, 1986; Barnett et al., 1989; Appleby et al., 1991; Hoofs, 1993) there still is discussion on its consequences for post weaning performance and health. One of the reasons for this lack in agreement is the high variability in creep feed intake between and within litters (Pajor et al., 1991; Barnett et al., 1989). From Dutch studies on creep intake per litter it may be concluded that the intake per litter also varies considerable.

Bruininx et al. (submitted) assessed the effects of pre weaning creep feed consumption on post weaning individual feed intake and performance of group-housed weanling piglets. According to the method of Barnett et al. (1989), Bruininx et al. (submitted) added 1% chromic oxide to a commercial pelleted (2 mm) creep feed (13.7 g/kg ileal digestible lysine and 12.7 MJ/kg Net Energy) as an index of feed consumption during the sucking period. A green colour of the feces, due to the presence of chromic oxide, indicated that the pig had eaten creep feed (Barnett et al., 1989). On d 18, 22, and 27 after birth fecal samples were taken using fecal loops as described by Barnett et al. (1989). Piglets that showed green coloured feces at all three sampling moments were designated as "eaters". Piglets that never showed green coloured feces were designated as "non-eaters". At weaning (28 d after birth), "eaters", "non-eaters" and "non-fed" pigs were selected based on gender and body weight and housed in pens equipped with IVOG®- feeding stations for weanling piglets in order to measure individual feed intake (Bruininx et al., 2001c). Each pen contained eaters, non-eaters and non-fed piglets. The average performance traits for the three creep feed types are presented in table 2 (Bruininx et al., submitted). Averaged over the first 13 days after weaning, eaters

Table 2. Performance of weanling piglets as affected by creep feed characterisation during nursing (Bruininx et al., submitted).

	Eaters	Non-eaters	Non fed	Sign.[a]
Number of piglets	22	22	22	
Day 0-13				
ADFI (g/d)	267	224	209	#
ADG (g/d)	188[b]	141[c]	137[c]	*
Day 0-34				
ADFI (g/d)	539	484	502	n.s.
ADG (g/d)	377[b]	314[c]	321[c]	*

[a] Significance: n.s. = P > 0.1; # = P < 0.1; * = P < 0.05
[bc] Means within a row with different superscript are significantly different (P<0.05)

tended to eat more (P < 0.1) than the non-fed pigs whereas the averaged daily feed intake (ADFI) of the non-eaters was intermediate. Moreover, averaged daily gain (ADG) of the eaters was higher (P<0.05) than ADG of Non eaters and Non-fed pigs. Averaged over the total 34-day period the effect of creep feed intake on post weaning ADFI was less pronounced (P=0.11), whereas ADG of the eaters was the highest (P<0.05). Furthermore, the individual feed intake data showed that about 50% of the eaters started eating within 4 hours after weaning whereas 50% of the non-eaters and non-fed piglets needed 6.7 and 6.9 hours respectively.

The results of Bruininx et al. (submitted) show that creep feed intake by suckling pigs stimulates early post weaning feed intake as well as post weaning performance. However, the minimum amount of creep feed that a piglet has to eat prior to weaning to obtain an advantage in post-weaning performance remains to be established.

Stimulation of the intake of creep feed

Creep feeding is supposed to prevent pigs from developing PWS. Piglets that consumed at least 600 g of solid feed during a lactation period of 28 days had improved feed intake and performance after weaning (English 1980). Several experiments have been conducted to stimulate creep feed intake of young piglets. One of the methods used for stimulating feed intake is interrupted suckling. This is a management technique by which piglets are separated from the sow during a number of hours every day during the second part of the lactation. In one Dutch experiment (Plagge et al 1998) interrupted suckling did not lead to a higher consumption of creep feed. However, in another Dutch experiment (Kuller et al 2000) the feed intake of the piglets of the interrupted suckling group was 708 g during lactation versus 320 g for the control-group. The authors of the first study suggest that the lack of result was due to stress of piglets in the interrupted suckling group who were in the same room as the piglets that had free access to the sow.

5.4.3. Weaning strategy

In 1998, Dutch legislation on pig welfare was revised, allowing more space for weaning and fattening pigs. Furthermore, it stated that pigs should only be mixed from birth to one week after weaning. After initial mixing it is only allowed to maintain or split up an intact group of piglets. Group composition (e.g., mixing of littermates), gender and body weight can affect social interactions, early feed intake, and performance of weanling piglets (Pluske et al., 1996c; Mahan et al., 1998; Bruininx et al., 2001b). According to Pluske and Williams (1996) mixing unacquainted piglets at weaning does increase aggression but this does not necessarily lead to a decrease in performance. These findings are partly in accordance with the results of Bruininx et al. (2001b). These workers assessed the effects of body weight distribution within groups (homogeneous vs. heterogeneous) and body weight class on performance and individual feed intake characteristics. Homogeneous groups (10-11 pigs) consisted of pigs of the same body weight class whereas heterogeneous groups (10-11 pigs) consisted of pigs of all three body weight classes (light- vs. middle- vs. heavy weight). In accordance with Pluske and Williams (1996c), this study indicated that BW distribution within groups has only limited effects on pig performance. A homogeneous versus heterogeneous group composition improved gain to feed ratio but did not affect ADG and ADFI (Table 3). However, during the first days after weaning the amount of feed consumed during the final 24 h after the first recorded feed intake (= initial feed intake) was affected by an interaction between BW distribution and BW class. Compared with their counterpart pigs in heterogeneous groups, heavy-weight pigs (9.3 kg) in homogeneous groups showed a 57 percent lower initial feed intake whereas that of middle-weight (7.9 kg) and light-weight (6.7 kg) pigs was not affected by weight distribution within groups (Bruininx et al., 2001b).

Table 3. Growth performance[a] of weanling piglets as affected by body weight distribution within groups and body weight class (Bruininx et al., 2001b).

Period	Weight distribution within groups		Body weight class		
	Heterogeneous	Homogeneous	Light	Middle	Heavy
Number of pigs	94	92	65	61	60
Weaning weight, kg	8.0	8.0	6.7[c]	7.9[d]	9.3[e]
Day 0-13					
ADFI, g/d[b]	176	179	168	175	190
ADG, g/d	118	120	122	117	121
Gain:Feed, kg/kg	0.43	0.61	0.73[c]	0.57[cd]	0.26[d]
Day 14-34					
ADFI, g/d[2]	493	489	452[c]	486[c]	535[d]
ADG, g/d	320	321	298[c]	320[cd]	345[d]
Gain:Feed, kg/kg	0.65[c]	0.67[d]	0.67	0.66	0.65

[a] Data are given as estimated means
[b] ADFI values are based on feed intake registration by feeding stations.
[c,d,e] Within a row and within a factor means without a common superscript differ (P < 0.05)

5.5. Pre- and post weaning diets: formulation

5.5.1. Creep feed

Using video-recording in combination with electronic monitoring of the amount of creep feed in the dispenser, Fraser et al. (1994) monitored the creep feeding behaviour and performance of piglets fed one of two different diets: a high-complexity creep diet without soybean meal or a low-cost alternative using soybean as the main protein source. Both diets were fed two weeks before and two weeks after weaning. Pigs fed the high-complexity diet consumed more creep feed, tended to gain more during the week before weaning, and converted feed more efficiently and also gained more weight in the two weeks after weaning (Table 4). However, even with the high-complexity diet, creep feed intake varied widely between littermates.

Table 4. Mean (+ SEM) performance of litters on a high- (n=12) or low-complexity diet (n=12) before and after weaning at 28 d. (Fraser et al., 1994).

	High complexity diet	Low complexity diet
Creep feeding before weaning (g/d)		
Intake, week 3	11 ± 2.5[a]	5 ± 1.0[b]
Intake, week 4	44 ± 9.3[a]	18 ± 5.4[b]
Gain before weaning (g/d)		
week 3	220 ± 6	211 ± 7
week 4	263 ± 7	232 ± 6
Gain after weaning (g/d)		
week 5: day 1	-129 ± 19	-98 ± 24
day 2-4	269 ± 10[a]	137 ± 11[b]
day 5-7	258 ± 9[a]	115 ± 11[b]
week 6	463 ± 9[a]	315 ± 12[b]

[ab] Means within a row with different superscript are significantly different (P<0.05)

In order to stimulate the feed intake in the young piglet, Edge et al. (2000) manipulated the physical form of the pre- and post weaning diet with regard to pellet size. In a 2x3 factorial study, all litters received either a pellet 1.8 mm or 5.0 mm in diameter in the farrowing house followed by each pen receiving either a 1.8m, 2.4 or 5.0 mm diameter pellet in the weaner accommodation. These authors found no significant differences between the treatments in terms of production data. However, pellet diameter did significantly affect feeding behaviour. The litters of piglets fed the 5.0 diameter pellet as a creep feed spent more time engaged in feeding related behaviour than litters receiving 1.8 mm pellet. It was concluded that while the presentation of the diet can attract the piglet to the feeder it does not improve feed intake. However, in practice feed companies claim that pre weaning feed intake can be stimulated by providing a 2 mm pellet. Moreover, the fat content of the creep diet as well as the hardness of the pellet may also affect the intake of creep feed by nursing piglets. Additionally, when the feed is mixed with water and provided, as a fresh porridge, practical findings suggest an improvement in feed intake.

5.5.2. Weaner diet

In general, the factor most limiting performance of the weaned pig is a limited energy intake. Newly weaned pigs, have a unique requirement for a diet of high nutrient density, high palatability and high digestibility (Thacker, 1999). Toplis and Tibble (1995) showed that feed intake of 10 kg piglets is positively correlated to diet digestibility. Therefore, only feedstuffs with a high digestibility should be used. Recently, Thacker (1999) reviewed recent research on the nutrient requirements of the weaned pigs. The following paragraph is partly based on this review.

5.5.3. Carbohydrate sources

Starch is the main energy source in weanling piglets diets. Coarseness of grinding, cooking and pelleting temperature influence starch digestibilily. Complex carbohydrates are utilised less efficiently by the weaned pig compared to simple carbohydrates such as lactose (Mahan and Newton, 1993). Therefore, products such as whey or lactose are widely utilised in diets formulated for (early) weaned pigs. However, a certain level of fermentable carbohydrates is seems to be needed for an optimal fermentation in the large intestine. Processed cereals are also considered as highly digestible carbohydrate sources in weaner diets. However, extreme processing also makes starch more available for micro organisms in the small intestine and may lead to digestion disorders and diarrhoea.
The increasing insight on the potentially beneficial activities of the gastrointestinal microflora (colonization resistence; Hentges, 1992) and the increasing concern on the use of anti microbial growth promoting agents have resulted in research on alternatives for in-feed antibiotics. It has been suggested that by the addition of certain non-digestible oligosaccharides (NDO) selectively stimulate the growth and/or activity of one or a limited number of bacteria and thus improve host health (Hidaka et al. 1985; Katta et al., 1993). Houdijk (1998) studied the prebiotic effects of two types of NDO in pig diets: frucooligosaccharides (FOS) and transgalactooligosaccharides (TOS). This author concluded that both NDO types had little effect on growth performance and nutrient digestion. Nevertheless, dietary FOS and TOS enhanced the precaecal saccharolytic activity, resulting in prebiotic effects. However, these effects were not maintained throughout the total large intestine, due to the fast rate of fermentation of FOS and TOS. Prebiotic carbohydrates which can be fermented throughout the total gastrointestinal tract, rather than only in the small intestine and/or proximal colon may result in prebiotic effects in (young) pigs.

5.5.4. Protein sources

Due to high amino acid requirements of the early-weaned pig not only for the increase in body-weight, but also for the increase in weight of the intestinal tissue, the inclusion of multiple protein sources in the weaner diet is necessary. However, quantification of particular nutrient requirements for growth and function of the gastro-intestinal tract has not been explored completely. Burrin (2000) reported that the gastrointestinal tissues utilize nearly 50% of dietary amino acid intake, and metabolise non-essential amino acids to a greater extent than essential amino acids. Moreover, the tissues derive a substantial proportion of their essential acid needs from the arterial circulation rather than from the diet.

However, weaner diets consist of lots of less digestible non-milk proteins. Non-milk-proteins could be considered as irritating or hypersensitivity inducing agents as investigated by several authors. For example, in the late eighties, it was suggested that dietary antigens could be responsible for damage of the intestinal wall caused by transient hypersensitivity (Miller et al, 1984). From the research work done by the group of Lallès (1993) it can be concluded that proteins from plant origin damage the wall of the small intestine. Factors in soybean other than the main ANF have been suggested to cause hypersensitivity reactions in the small intestine, leading to poor growth. By a combined heat and alcohol treatment, two proteins in soy (glycinin and β-conglycinin), can be removed. Feeding these heat- and-alcohol-treated soy protein to pigs weaned at 21 d resulted in improved weight gain, less frequent diarrhoea, longer villi in the small intestine, and lower eosinophil density in the duodenal mucosa than feed soy proteins treated with heat only (Dréau et al., 1994). Additionally, legume seeds contain anti-nutritional factors, which cause most of the damage (Zijlstra 1996).

Makkink et al. (1994) compared weaner diets with skimmed milk powder, soybean-protein concentrate, soybean meal, or fishmeal as protein sources in 28-day-old weaned pigs. No differences in weight and morphology of the small intestine were observed. However, dietary protein source affected trypsin and chymotrypsin activities in jejunal digesta. Dietary fishmeal resulted in low enzyme activities, whereas skimmed-milk powder and soybean-protein concentrate were associated with high enzyme activities.

Most diets for weanling piglets contain some combinations of skim milk, fish meal, whey protein concentrate, processed potato protein, heat treated soybean meal, and further processed soy products (soy concentrate or isolate). Until recently spray dried animal plasma (SDPP) was a highly recommended protein source in weaner diets. Summarizing 25 experiments on the inclusion of spray dried porcine plasma, Weaver et al. (cited by Thacker, 1999) concluded that on average daily gain had been improved by 39%, daily feed intake was increased by 32% and feed efficiency was improved by 5.4%. However, the mode of action of porcine plasma products is not completely clear yet. Van Dijk et al (2001) suggested that immunoglobulins that are present in SDPP are the cause of the improvement of post weaning piglet performance and health. Moreover, due to the European ban on the use of animal proteins in pig diets, the use of spray dried animal plasma products as well as blood meal products are not allowed. Whether spray dried porcine plasma and other animal protein products can be used in pig diets in the future or not was not known on the date of publication of these proceedings.

Van der Peet-Schwering and Binnendijk (2000) showed that from day 1 to 14 and from day 1 to 34 after weaning piglets receiving a diet with 3% protein from protein-rich whey-concentrate had the same performance as the piglets that were fed a diet with wheypowder + animal plasma. These authors concluded that whey concentrate can be a good alternative for wheypowder + animal plasma in weaner diets. It is interesting to note that in this experiment there were no significant differences in performance between the above mentioned diets and third experimental diet with only protein sources of plant origin.

Potato protein is also considered to be a high quality protein source for weanling piglets. In the past, only limited amounts of potato protein (< 4%) were included in weaner diets due to a low palatability and high content of glyco-alcaloids (Smith et al., 1994). Plagge and Van der Peet-Schwering (1996) concluded that the performance of piglets fed a diet with a new type of processed (reduction of glyco-alcaloids) potato protein (5% inclusion level) was similar to the performance of piglets fed a diet with 3% milk protein (milk powder and low lactose whey powder).

5.5.5. *Fat sources*

A wide variety of fats and oils has been employed by various workers to study the effect of fat supplementation to swine diets. The response of pigs to the addition of dietary fat is affected by interactions between different fatty acids of the diet (Bayley and Lewis, 1965), the relationship between energy content and amino acids (Allee et al., 1971), the age of the pigs (Cera et al., 1988c) and mainly the concentration and composition of the dietary fat (Hamilton and McDonald, 1969; Cera et al., 1988b). Mountzouris et al. (1999) concluded that dietary fats formulated by combination of various animal fats and vegetable oils to resemble the fatty acid composition of sow milk fat can be effectively used as supplementary fats for weaner diets. In practice lard, coconut, soybean oil or mixtures are widely used for weaner diets in order to get a higher energy level per kg diet. Furthermore, fat can improve the taste and feed intake directly after weaning. It is important that high quality fat sources are used (smell, no oxidation, low free fatty acids). Moreover, the level of linoleic acid and the ratio of omega-3/omega-6 fatty acids in the diet seem to affect health and performance of the weaned piglet.

5.5.6. *Flavours*

In order to stimulate post weaning feed intake, the use of feed flavours in weaner diets is widely spread. However, very few studies have demonstrated a consistent improvement in feed intake or growth rate as a result of the inclusion of feed flavour in de weaner diet (Pluske 1993). A total of 129 flavours or flavour combinations were tested by McLaughlin et al. (1983). Two ("cheesy" and "sweet, molasses caramel") of five by weanling piglets highly preferred flavours were used in a performance trial. Compared with a non-flavoured diet, both flavours did not increase feed intake or growth rate.

5.6. Practical considerations: feed and water provision

5.6.1. Water

Gill et al. (1989) showed that it could take more than a week for the pig to restore its daily fluid intake to the equivalent of that on the day before weaning. Thus the pig is seriously dehydrated for a prolonged period of time. Therefore, it is also important to encourage pigs to drink following weaning. Drinker design and positioning can both contribute to the acquisition of water post-weaning and can affect both piglet performance and water use. Where nipple drinkers are provided, the positioning of the drinker is most important. Consumption can be inhibited if the drinker is placed at the incorrect height and angle and if the drinker is incorrectly placed in the pen (Brooks, 1999). Increasing the water delivery rate from 175 to 450 ml/min increased daily intake by 12.5% and daily gain by 17.6% (Barber, 1989; Table 5).

In a study by Bokma and Duijf (1988) a bite nipple drinker (300-400 ml/min) and a drinking bowl (nipple inside: 500 ml/min) were considered to be suitable water supply systems for weanling piglets. To avoid spillage the bite nipple drinker as well as the drinking bowl should be positioned such that the piglets are forced to stand straight in front of them while drinking. The drinking bowl minimises water losses, but contamination of drinking water may occur.
By using a dry feed hopper with a drink nipple in the trough (semi-liquid feeder) the use of water can be reduced without a loss in piglet performance (Plagge, 1990).

5.6.2. Feeding systems

In the past, dry feeding systems for weaner pigs housed in groups of about 10 animals, could be divided in to two categories. Long throughs made it possible that all pigs could eat at the same time whereas ad lib hoppers provided eating space for only some

Table 5. Effect of flow rate of water on weaner pig performance (3-6 weeks) (Barber, 1989).

	Water delivery rate (ml/minute)			
	175	350	450	700
Time spent drinking (min)	4.46[a]	2.97[b]	2.93[b]	2.32[b]
Water used (L/d)	0.78[a]	1.04[b]	1.32[c]	1.63[d]
Feed intake (g/d)	303[a]	323[b]	341[c]	347[c]
Daily gain (g/d)	210[a]	235[b]	250[c]	247[c]
Feed conversion ratio	1.48	1.39	1.37	1.42

[abcd] Means without a common superscript differ (P<0.05)

pigs. Long throughs allow social facilitation and permit continuation of the group-feeding behaviour that the pigs practise pre weaning. According to Brooks (1999) the practice of feeding discrete meals in long throughs can reduce agonistic behaviour around the feeder and can also reduce the chances of submissive pigs being kept away from the feed. However, in a 14 d study by Plagge (unpublished data) no effects of the number of eating places (2 vs. 9) on the performance of restrictively fed (meal) weaner pigs were found. Because of limited space availability many pig producers prefer to use ad libitum feeding systems. The merit of an ad libitum feed dispenser is likely to be affected by its position within the pen and its relationship to the drinker and also the pigs lysing area (Brooks, 1999).

Additionally, the results of Bruininx et al. (2001b) suggested that illumination of the nursery room stimulates early feed intake by weanling piglets. Using artificial lighting from 0700 to 1900 each day, these authors found that after weaning the majority of the pigs start eating when lights were on compared to control group? (Figure 2).

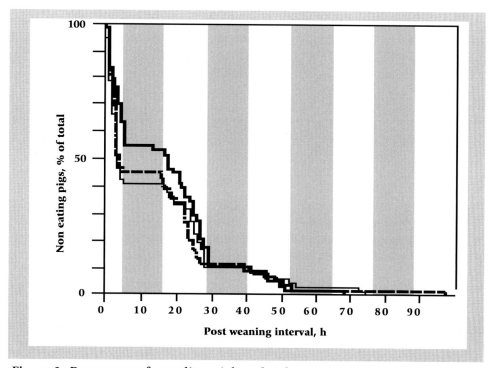

Figure 2. Percentage of weanling piglets that has not eaten after weaning as a function of post weaning interval (mean = 15.4 h; SD = 1.38 h). Curves are given for light (——), middle (- - -) and heavy (——) weanling piglets. The dark periods are indicated by shaded bars (Bruininx et al., 2001b).

5.7. Conclusions

The aim of this paper was to review the mechanisms by which feed and feeding strategy influence the health status of the gastro-intestinal tract of the pig. Health problems that occasionally occur in swineherds are difficult to prevent by vaccination, as passive immunity lasts as long as the pigs suckle and active immunity is not developed until 4 - 7 weeks of age. Health problems caused by environmental agents like *E. coli* and *S. suis* can be suppressed by low pH of the stomach, intact mucosal wall, well-equipped digestive system and a stable flora in the large intestine. A continuous supply of nutrients (energy) on gut level seems very important to maintain villous architecture as well as the digestive capacity. Therefore, early post weaning feed intake has to be stimulated in order to maintain health and performance of the weanling pig. Providing nursing piglets with a creep feed seems to be a usefull strategy to stimulate post weaning feed intake and growth. Additionally, the provision of a highly digestible diet after weaning, together with optimal husbandry and hygienic conditions will help the weaned piglet to maintain health and performance during the first week after weaning.

5.8. References

Allee, G.L., D.H. Barker, G.A. Leveille, 1971. Fat utilization and lipogenesis in the young pig. Journal of Nutrition, 101, 1415-1421.

Alpers, D.H., J. Binder, D.O. Castell, D.K. Podolsky, and J.D. Wood, 1992 in: The undergraduate teaching project in gastroenterology and liver disease. Milner-fenwick Inc. Timonium, Maryland, USA, 27

Appleby, M.C. , E.A. Pajor, and D. Fraser, 1991. Effects of management options on creep feeding by piglets. Animal Production 53, 361-366.

Barber, J., P.H. Brooks, and J.L. Carpenter 1989. The effect of water delivery rate on voluntary food intake, water use and performance of early-weaned pigs from 3 to 6 weeks of age. In:Frobes, J.M., M.A. Varley, and T.L.J. Lawrence (editors), The voluntary food intake of pigs: Occasional publication No. 13. British Society of Animal Production., Edinburgh, UK, pp. 103-104.

Bark, L.J., T.D.Crenshaw, V.D. Leibbrandt, 1986. The effect of meal intervals and weaning on feed intake of early weaned pigs. Journal of Animal Science 62, 1233-1239.

Barnett, K.L., E.T., Kornegay, C.R. Risley, M.D. Lindemann and G.G. Schurig, 1989.

Burrin, D.G., B.Stoll, J.B. van Goudoever and P.J.Reeds, 2000. In: Lindberg, J.E. and B.Ogle (editors) Proceedings of the 8th Symposium of Digestive physiology of Pigs published by CABI Publishing, Ch 19, 75-88

Characterisation of creep feed consumption and its subsequent effects on immune response, scouring index and performance of weanling pigs. Journal of Animal Science 67, 2698-2708.

Bayley, H.S., D. Lewis, 1965. The use of fats in pig feeding. II. The digestibility of various fats and fatty acids. Journal of Agricultural Science 64, 373-378.

Beachy, E.H., 1981. Bacterial adherence: adhesin-receptor interactions mediating the attachment of bacteria to mucosal surfaces. Journal of Infectious Diseases 143, 325-345

Berg, R.D., 1992 Translocation of enteric bacteria in health and disease. In: Gut-derived Infectious-Toxic Shock.Cottier H, R. Kraft (eds) Current Studies in Hematology and Transfusion, Basel, Karger. 59, 44-65

Bohl, E.H., 1979. Rotaviral diarrhea in pigs: Brief review. Journal of American Veterinary Medicine Association 174:613-615.

Bokma, S. and J.M. Duijf 1988. Drinkwatervoorzieningen voor gespeende biggen. Research Institute for Pig Husbandry, Raalte, The Netherlands, Research Report P1.25.

Bovee-Oudenhoven, I.M., Termont D.S., Heidt P.J., Van der Meer, R. 1997. Increasing the intestinal resistance of rats to the invasive pathogen *Salmonella enteritidis*: additive effects of dietary lactulose and calcium. Gut 40, 497-504.

Brooks, P.H., 1999. Strategies and methods for the allocation of food and water in the post-weaning period. Paper 5.4 presented to the 50th Meeting of the European Association of Animal Production, Zurich, August 22-26.

Brown, I.H., S. Done, D. Hanman, R.J. Higgins, S.C. Machey, and A. Courtenay, 1992. An outbreak of influenza in pigs. Veterinary Record 130, 166

Brown, P.J., B.G. Miller, C.R. Stokes, N.B. Blazquez and F.J. Bourne 1988. Histochemistry of mucins of pig intestinal secretory epithelial cells before and after weaning. Journal of Comparative Pathology 98, 313-323.

Bruininx, E.M.A.M., C.M.C. van der Peet-Schwering and J.W. Schrama. 2001a. Individual feed intake of group-housed weaned pigs and health status In: Varley, M.A. and J. Wiseman (editors), The Weaner Pig: Nutrition and Management. Published by CABI Publishing, Ch 6, 113-122.

Bruininx, E.M.A.M., C.M.C. van der Peet-Schwering, J.W. Schrama, P.F.G. Vereijken, P.C. Vesseur, H. Everts, L.A. den Hartog, and A.C. Beynen, 2001b. Individually measured feed intake characteristics and growth performance of group-housed weanling pigs: effects of sex, initial body weight, and body weight distribution within groups. Journal of Animal Science 79, 301-308.

Bruininx, E.M.A.M., C.M.C. van der Peet-Schwering, J.W. Schrama, P.C. Vesseur, H. Everts, and A.C. Beynen, 2001c The IVOG® feeding station: a tool for monitoring the individual feed intake of group-housed weanling pigs. Journal of Animal Physiology and Animal Nutrition, 85, 81-87.

Bruininx, E.M.A.M., G.P. Binnendijk, C.M.C. van der Peet-Schwering, J.W. Schrama, L.A. den Hartog, H. Everts, and A.C. Beynen. Effect of creep feed consumption on individual feed intake characteristics and performance of group housed weanling pigs. submitted.

Cera, E. G. Charlier, G. and A. Houvenaghel, 1988a. Effect of age, weaning and post weaning diet on small intestinal growth and jejunal morphology in young swine. Journal of Animal Science 66, 574-584.

Cera, K. R., D. C Mahan, G.A. Reinhart 1988b. Weekly digestibility of diets supplemented with corn oil, lard or tallow by weanling swine. Journal of Animal Science 66, 1438-1445.

Cera, K. R., D. C Mahan, G.A. Reinhart 1988c. Effects of dietary whey and corn oil on weanling pig performance and fat digestibility and nitrogen utilization. Journal of Animl Science, 66, 1438-1445.

Dréau, D. J.P. Lallès, V. Philouze-Romé, R. Toullec and H. Salmon, 1994. Lcoal and systemic immune responses to soybean protein ingestion in early weaned piglets. Journal of Animal Science, 72, 2090-2098.

Diemen, P.M. van, J.W. Schrama, W. van der Hel, M.W.A. Verstegen, and J.P.T.M. Noordhuizen, 1995. Effects of Atrophic Rhinitis and climatic environment on the performance of pigs. Livestock Production Science 43: 275.

Edge, H.L., J.A. Dalby, P. Rowlinson, M.A. Varley. In: The Weaner Pig, Book of Abstracts, BSAS Occasional Meeting, University of Nottingham, 5-7 September 2000.

English, P.R. 1980. Establishing the early weaned pig. Pig Veterinary Society Proceedings 29-37

Field, M. 1981. Secretion of small intestine. In: Johnson LR ed. Physiology of the gastrointestinal tract. New York, Raven Press 2:963-982.

Fraser, D., J.J.R. Feddes, and E.A. Pajor, 1994. The relationship between creep feeding behavior of piglets and adaptation to weaning: Effect of diet quality. Canadian Journal of Animal Science 74, 1-6.

Gaskins, H., and K.W. Kelley 1995. Immunology and neonatal mortality. In: The Neonatal Pig Development and Survival. Varley, M.A. (ed). CAB International, Wallingford, Oxon, UK

Gill, B.P. 1989. Water use by pigs managed under various conditions of housing, feeding and nutrition. Ph.D. dissertation, University of Plymouth, UK.

Gentry, J.L., J.W.G.M. Swinkels, M.D. Lindemann, and J.W. Schrama, 1997. Effect of hemoglobin and immunisation status on energy metabolism of weanling pigs. Journal of Animal Science 75:1032-1040.

Hall, G.A., T.F. Byrne, 1989. Effects of age and diet on small intestinal structure and function in gnotobiotic pigs. Research in Veterinary Science: 47:387-392.

Hamilton, R., B. McDonald, 1969. Effects of dietary fat source nad level on utilization of fat and the composition of fecal lipids on the young pigs. Journal of Nutrition, 97, 33-41.

Hampson, D.J., 1986. Influence of creep feeding and dietary intake after weaning on malabsorption and occurence of diarrhoea in the newly weaned pig. Research in Veterinary Science: 41:63-69.

Hampson, D.J., M. Hinton, and D.E. Kidder, 1985. Coliform numbers in the stomach and small intestine of healthy pigs following weaning at three weeks of age. Journal of Comparative Pathology 95 :353-362.

Hampson, D.J. and D.E. Kidder, 1986. Influence of creep feeding and weaning on brush border enzyme activities in the piglet small intestine. Research in Veterinary Science 40, 24-31.

Hentges D.J., 1992. Gut flora and disease resistence. In: Probiotics. The scientific basis Fuller. R. (Ed.). Chapman & Hall Ltd. London, 87-110.

Hidaka, H., T. Eida, T. Hashimoto, and T. Nakazawa, 1985. Feeds for domestic anaimals and methods for breeding them. Eur. Pat. Appl. 133547A2: 1-14 .

Higgins, R. and M.Gottschalk, 1999. Streptococcal diseases. In: Diseases of Swine, B.E. Straw, S. D'Allaire, W.L. Mengeling, D.J. Taylor (ed) 8th ed. Iowa State University Press, Ames, Iowa 50014. 563

Hoofs, A. 1993. Wel of niet bedrijfsmatig bijvoeren van zogende biggen met vast voer. Research Institute for Pig Husbandry, Sterksel, Research report P1.97.

Houdijk, J. 1998. Effects of non-digestible oligosaccharides in young pig diets. Ph.D. dissertation. Department of Animal Sciences, Animal Nutrition Group, Wageningen Agricultural University, The Netherlands.

Katta, Y., K. Ohkuma, M. Satouchi, R. Takahashi, and T. Yamamoto, 1993. Feed for Livestock. Eur. Pat. Appl. 0549478A1, 1-14.

Hoofs, A. 1993. Wel of niet bedrijfsmatig bijvoeren van zogende biggen met vast voer. Research Institute for Pig Husbandry, Sterksel, Research report P1.97.

Kelly, D., J.A. Smyth, and K.J. McCracken, 1991. Digestive development in the early-weaned pig. II. Effect of level of food intake on digestive enzyme activity during the immediate post-weaning period. British Journal of Nutrition 65, 181-188.

Kenworthy R., 1976. Observations on the effects of weaning in the young pig. Clinical and histopathological studies of intestinal function and morphology. Research in Veterinary Science 2,1, 69-75.

Kuller W.I., H.M.G. Van Beers-Schreurs, N.M. Soede, M.A.M. Taverne, J.H.M.Verheijden, and B. Kemp, 2000 Interrupted suckling: effects on growth and feedintake of the piglets and reproductive performance of the sow. MSc Thesis Utrecht University. The Netherlands.

Lallès, J.P., H. Salmon, N.P.M. Bakker, and G.H. Tolman 1993. Effect of dietary antigens on health, performance and immune system of calves and piglets. In: Recent Advances of Research in Antinutritional Factors of Legume Seeds. In: Van der Poel, A.F.B., J. Huisman and H.S. Saini (editors), Proceedings of the Second International Workshop on Antinutritional Factors in legume seeds. Wageningen Pers, The Netherlands, pp. 253-270.

Le Dividich, J. and P. Herpin, 1994. Effects of climatic conditions on the performance, metabolism and health status of weaned pigs: A review. Livestock Production Science 38, 79-90.

Lecce, J.G., R.K. Balsbaugh, D.A.Clare, and M.W. King, 1982. Rotavirus and hemolytic enteropathogenic Escherichia coli in weanling diarrhea of pigs. Journal of Clinical Microbiology 16: 715-723.

Lindemann, M.D., S.G. Cornelius, S.M. El Kandelgy, R.M. Moser, J.E. Pettigrew, 1986. Effect of age, weaning and diet on digestive enzyme levels in the piglet. Journal of Animal Science, 69, 1298-1307.

Mahan, D. C. , G. L. Cromwell, R. C. Ewan, C. R. Hamilton, and J. T. Yen. 1998. Evaluation of the feeding of a phase 1 nursery diet to three-week-old pigs of two weaning weights. Journal of Animal Science, 76: 578-583.

Mahan, D.C and E. A. Newton, 1993. Evaluation of feed grains with dried skim milk and added carbohydrate sources on weanling pig performance. Journal of Animal Science, 69, 1397-1402.

Makkink, C. A., 1993. Of piglets, dietary proteins, and pancreatic proteases. Ph.D. dissertation. Department of Animal Nutrition, Wageningen Agricultural University, The Netherlands.

Makkink, C.A., G.P. Neglescu, Q. Guixin, and M.W.A. Verstegen, 1994. Effects of dietary protein on feed intake, growth, pancreatic enzyme activities and jejunal morphology in newly-weaned piglets. British Journal of Nutrition, 72, 353-368.

McCracken, B.A., H.R. Gaskins, P.J. Ruwe-Kaiser, K.C. Klasing, and J.E. Jewell, 1995. Diet-Dependent and Diet-Independent Metabolic Responses Underlie Growth Stasis of Pigs at Weaning. Journal of Nutrition, 125, 2838-2845.

McLaughlin, C.L., C.A. Baile, L.L. Buckholtz and S.K. Freeman, 1983. Preferred flavours and performance of weaner pigs. Journal of Animal Science, 56, 1287-1293.

Miller, B.G., T.J. Newby, C.R. Stokes, and F.J. Bourne, 1984. Influence of diet on postwea ning malabsorption and diarrhoea in the pig. Research in Veterinary Science 36:187-193.

Moon, H.K., I.K. Han, H.K. Parmentier, and J.W. Schrama, 1997. Effects of a cell mediated immune response on energy metabolism in weanling piglets. In: McCracken, K., E.F. Unsworth, and A.R.G. Wylie (editors.) Proceedings 14th Symposium on Energy Metabolism of Farm Animals. CAB International, Wallingford, U.K. pp 143-146.

Mountzouris, K. C., K. Fegeros, G. Papadopoulos, 1999. Utilization of fats based on the composition of sow milk fat in the diet of weanling pigs. Animal Feed Science and Technology, 77, 115-124.

Nabuurs, M.J.A., A. Hoogendoorn, E.J. van der Molen, A.L.M. Osta, 1993. Villus height and crypt depth in weaned and unweaned pigs, reared under various circumstances in the Netherlands. Research in Veterinary Science 55:78-84

Nabuurs, M.J., A. Hoogendoorn,and F.G. van Zijderveld, 1994. Effects of weaning and enterotoxigenic Escherichia coli on net absorption in the small intestine of pigs. Research in Veterinary Science 56(3):379-385

Nielsen, N.O. Edema Disease. In: Leman AD, Straw B, Glock RD et al. eds. Diseases of Swine. Ames Iowa: Iowa State University Press 1986;528-40.

Niewold, T.A., G.J. van Essen, M.J.A. Nabuurs, N. Stockhofe-Zurwieden, and J. van der Meulen 2000. A review of porcine pathophysiology: a different approach to disease. Veterinary Quarterly 22:209-212

NRC. Nutrition requirements of swine. 10th revised edition. National Academy Press, Washington, DC. NRC, 1998

Pajor, E.A., D. Fraser, and D.L. Kramer, 1991. Consumption of solid food by suckling pigs: individual variation and relation to weight gain. Applied Animal Behaviour Science 32, 139-155.

Parsons, D.S. 1968. In : Code C.F and W. Heidel (editors) published by the American Physiological Society, Washington. Handbook of Physiology, section 6 : Alimentary Canal, volume III Intestinal absorption. Pp 1177-1216

Plagge, G. 1990. Vergelijking van droogvoerbak en brijbak voor gespeende biggen. Research Institute for Pig Husbandry, Raalte, The Netherlands, Research report P1.56.

Plagge, J.G. and C.M.C. van der Peet-Schwering, 1996. Aardappeleiwit (Protamyl® PF and Protastar®) in voer voor gespeende biggen. Research Insititute for Pig Husbandry, Rosmalen, The Netherlands, Research report P1.157

Plagge, J.G. and Van der Peet-Schwering, 1998. Het tijdelijk spenen van biggen. Praktijkonderzoek varkenshouderij, proefverslag P.4.32

Pluske, J.R. 1993. Psychological and nutritional stress in pigs at weaning: production parameters, the stress response, and histology and biochemistry of the small intestine. pp 21-22. Ph.D. Thesis. University of Western Australia.

Pluske, J.R. and I.H. Williams, 1996. The influence of feeder type and the method of group allocation at weaning on voluntary food intake and growth in piglets. Animal Science, 62, 115-120.

Pluske, J. R., I.H. Williams, and H.X. Aherne, 1996a Maintenance of villous height and crypt depth in piglets by providing continuous nutrition after weaning. Animal Science 62, 131-144.

Pluske, J. R., I.H. Williams, and H.X. Aherne, 1996b. Villous height and crypt depth in piglets in response to increases in the intake of cows'milk after weaning. Animal Science 62, 145-158.

Pluske, J.R., M.J. Thompson, C.S. Atwood, P.H. Bird, I.H. Williams, and P.E. Hartmann, 1996c. Maintenance of villous height and crypt depth, and enhancement of disaccharide digestion and monosaccharide absorption, in piglets fed on cows' whole milk after weaning. British Journal of Nutrition 76, 409-422.

Porter, P. 1986 Immune system. In: Leman, A.D. (ed) Diseases of Swine, 6th edition Iowa State University Press, Ames, pp 44-57

Rerat, A, M. Fiszlewicz, P. Herpin and M. Durand 1985. Measurements of the appearance of volatile fatty acids in the portal vein during digestion in conscious pigs. Current Research Of Academic Science III, 300(12):467-470

Schumer, W. and P.R. Erve, 1975. Circ. Shock,2,109.

Sijben, J.W.C., P.N.A. van Vugt, J.W.G.M. Swinkels, H.K. Parmentier, and J.W. Schrama, 1998. Energy metabolism of immunised weanling pigs is not affected by dietary nucleotides. Journal of Animal Physiology and Animal. Nutrition. 79:153-161.

Smith, J.W., B.T. Richert, R.D. Goodband, J.L. Nelssen, M.D. Tokach, L.J. Kats, K.Q. Owen and S.S. Dritz, 1994. Evaluation of potato protein in starter pig diets. Swine Day, Kansas State University. Kansas, USA.

Smith, M.W.,1984. Effect of postnatal development and weaning upon the capacity of pig intestinal villi to transport alanine. Journal of Agricultural Science Cambridge 102:625-633.

Smith, H.W., and S. Halls. 1967. Studies on Escherichia coli enterotoxin. Journal of Pathology and Bacteriology 93 :531-543.

Solz,A. and F. Ponz, 1947. A new method for the study of intestinal absorption. Review Espanol Fisiologica 3:207-211

Stokes, C.R. and J.F. Bourne, 1989. Mucosal immunity. In: Halliwel, R.E.W. (ed). Veterinary Clinical Immunology. Harcourt Brace Jovanovich Inc., Philadelphia, 164-192

Svendsen J. 1974. Enteric Escherichia coli diseases in weaned pigs. Nordish Veterinary Medicine 2 6:226-238.

Tasman-Jones C., R. Owen, and A.L. Jones 1982. The effect of dietary fibre compo nents on the morphology of the small intestine of the rat. In: Robinson JWL, Dowling RH and Riecken EO eds. Mechanisms of intestinal adaptation. Lancaster: Raven Press 169-171.

Terpstra, J.I., 1958. Hemolytische colibacterien als oorzaak van ziekten bij het varken. Tijdschrift voor Diergeneeskunde 83:1078.

Thacker, P.A., 1999. Nutritional requirements of early weaned pigs: A review. Pig News and Information, 20, 2, 55N-58N.

Ti money, J.F. 1950.Oedema disease of swine. Veterinary Record 62:748-756.

Toplis, P. and S. Tibble, 1995. Appetite management of the pig. Beyond diet formulation. In: Proceedings of the 1995 Saskatchewan Pork Industry Symposium, 23-33, Saskatoon, Saskatchewan.

Tzipori, S., D. Chandler, T. Makin, and M. Smith. 1980 Escherichia coli and rotavirus infections in four-week-old gnotobiotic pigs fed milk or dry food. Australian Veterinary Journal 56 :279-284.

Ussing, H.H., and K. Zerahn, 1951. Active transport of sodium as the source of electric current in the short-circuited isolated frog skin. Acta physiologica Scandinavica 23;110-127.

Van Beers-Schreurs, H.M.G., L. Vellenga, Th. Wensing, and H.J. Breukink 1992. The pathogenesis of the post-weaning syndrome in pigs; a review. Veterinary Quarterly 14:29-34

Van Beers-Schreurs, H.M.G., M.J.A. Nabuurs, L. Vellenga, H.J. Kalsbeek-van der Valk, Th. Wensing, and H.J. Breukink, 1998a. Weaning and the weanling diet influnece the villous height and crypt depth in the small intestine of pigs and alter the concentrations of short-chain fatty acids in the large intestine and blood. Journal of Nutrition 128:947-953

Van Beers-Schreurs, H.M.G., M.J.A. Nabuurs, L. Vellenga, Th. Wensing, and H.J. Breukink, 1998b. Role of the large intestine in the pathogenesis of diarrhoea in weaned pigs. American Journal of Veterinary Research 59:696-703

Van Dijk, A.J., Everts, H., Nabuurs, M.J.A., Margry, R.J.C.F., & Beynen, A.C. 2001a. Growth performance of weanling pigs fed spray-dried animal plasma: a review. Livest. Prod. Sci. 68, 263-274.

Van der Peet-Schwering, C.M.C. and G.P. Binnendijk, 2000. Effect van eiwitbron in speenvoer op de technische resultaten en gezondheid van biggen. Research Institute for Pig Husbandry, Rosmalen, The Netherlands, Research report P1.243.

Van der Waaij, D., J.M. Berghuis de Vries, and J.E.C. Lekkerkerk van der Wees, 1971. Colonization resistance of the digestive tract in conventional and antibiotic treated mice. Journal of Hygienic Camb 69:405-411

Vellenga L. 1989. Intestinal permeability in pigs and rats. PhD Thesis State University Utrecht, the Netherlands.

Windsor, R.S. 1977. Meningitis in pigs caused by *Streptococcus suis* Type II. Veterinary Record 101:378-379

Worsaae, H., and M. Schmidt, 1980. Plasma cortisol and behaviour in early weaned piglets. Acta Veterinaria Scandinavica 21: 640-657.

Zijlstra, R.T., 1996. Physiological responses of the small intestine to nutritional factors and rotavirus infection afflicting young pigs. Ph.D dissertation, University of Illinois at Urbana-Champaign, Urbana, Illinois, USA.

6. The interactions between feed (components) and *Eimeria* infections in poultry health

Suzan H.M. Jeurissen[1] and Bert Veldman[2]
[1] *ID-Lelystad, P.O. Box 65, 8200 AB Lelystad, The Netherlands*
[2] *Institute for Animal Nutrition 'De Schothorst', P.O.Box 533, 8200 AM Lelystad, The Netherlands*

Introduction

World-wide, the consumption of poultry products still increases yearly; in 1998 the production of eggs was 48 million tons and the production of chicken meat exceeded 51 million tonnes (Watt Poultry Year Book, 1999). With the growing numbers of commercially held birds also the numbers increase of birds at risk of getting infected with pathogens, like bacteria, viruses and parasites.

Intestinal coccidiosis has become an important disease of poultry and livestock throughout the world, and in the Netherlands alone it causes approximately DFl 20 million (US\$ 13 million) in economic losses each year. Coccidiosis is caused by various species of *Eimeria* (phylum Apicomplexa of the protozoan parasites), who live out most of their lifecycle intracellularly. Coccidiosis is transmitted among animals, especially those kept in massive groups and in confinement pens, by oocysts released in the faeces of infected animals. The oocysts are resistant to climatic changes and can remain infectious for long periods.

In view of the economic importance of poultry, much effort is generated to protect the birds from being infected by improving their innate and adaptive defence, for instance, by adjusting feed and management conditions or by using vaccines.

6.1. Infection with *Eimeria* species

At least seven *Eimeria* species that effect chickens have been described and all 7 species occur in most European countries upon careful examination (Shirley et al., 1990; Williams et al., 1996). The life cycles of *Eimeria* species occur both outside (exogenous stages) and inside the host (endogenous stages). In figure 1, a schematic overview of the various stages of infection is given.

Oocysts are the exogenous stages of *Eimeria* and they are shed in the faeces of infected chickens. These environmentally resistant oocysts undergo sporogony outside the chicken. Sporogony is the process by which a one-celled zygote within the oocyst wall undergoes a series of divisions to form sporozoites, which are contained within

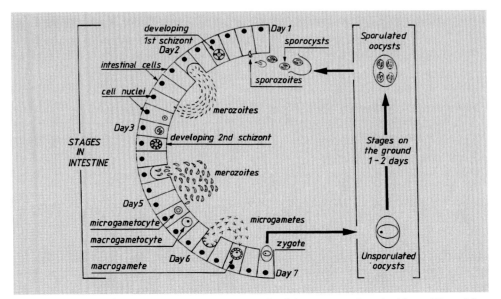

Figure 1. Life cycle of *Eimeria tenella*, typical of the genus *Eimeria* (from Vervelde, 1995b).

sporocysts. Only sporulated oocysts, those containing fully formed sporozoites, are infective to the chicken. After being ingested, the sporulated oocyst undergoes the process of excystation, the release of infective sporozoites. During excystation the oocyst wall is broken by the grinding process in the gizzard and the sporocysts are released. The release of sporozoites is caused by pancreatic enzymes and bile salts. Once free in the lumen, the motile sporozoites actively penetrate the intestinal epithelium.

Most *Eimeria* species have a characteristic site of invasion. In the chicken these locations are so characteristic that they are often used as diagnostic features of the individual species. For example, *Eimeria acervulina* parasitizes the duodenum, *E. maxima* the jejunum and ileum, and *E. tenella* the ceca. The ceca are two blind sacs appended to the junction of ileum and colon. Although Joyner (1982) suggested that the interval between the ingestion of oocysts and the release of sporozoites may be related to site specificity, it now appears that certain properties of the invasion site itself, such as secreted molecules, play a role in site specific development (Vervelde et al., 1993). Some species, such as *E. brunetti* and *E. praecox*, develop at the villus tips, the site of invasion, while others travel within the mucosa to the crypt epithelial cells where they develop further. Once within the crypt epithelium, sporozoites become rounded and transform into trophozoites, which undergo schizogony or merogony (formation of merozoites), the asexual proliferation phase. The merozoites are then released in the gut lumen, where they infect epithelial cells close to those from which they emerge and form additional schizont generations. After two to five schizont generations, gametogony (the formation of gametes), the sexual proliferation phase, occurs. During this phase, merozoites enter cells and develop into male microgametocytes or female macrogametocytes. A macrogametocyte is fertilised by a microgametocyte to form a zygote, which forms an environmentally resistant oocyst wall. The oocyst is released from its host cell and shed into the environment, where the process of sporogony occurs after which a new host can be infected. The time between the ingestion of sporulated oocysts and the appearance of first unsporulated oocysts in the faeces, that is the prepatent time, is constant and lasts four to seven days. The proliferation of the parasites extensively destroys the intestinal epithelium, starting for E. tenella on day 3 and peaking on day 5 post infection. The intestinal wall becomes greatly swollen, bloody diarrhoea occurs, and fibrin clots appear in the faeces.

6.2. Effect of *Eimeria* infection on bird health and performance

The host metabolic response to an infection is characterised by diverse alterations, which have been clearly described. The general pattern is fever, anorexia, a higher nutrient requirement, a lower digestibility, and a shift of the balance between anabolism and catabolism to the latter (Keusch et al., 1986). Fever during an infection means an increase in metabolic rate by about 13 % per degree Celsius, resulting in higher energy requirements than usual at a time when the host is often anorexic. Since carbohydrate stores are inadequate to meet these needs, and lipid stores are not effectively used in the infected host, another source of energy is required. In most infections, this turns out to be gluconeogenesis, the production of glucose by the liver from amino acids precursors released from contractile proteins of muscle (catabolism).

An *Eimeria* infection of chicks causes in addition to the general aspect of an infection also damage of the intestinal tract with implications for nutrient digestion and absorption. The combined effects of anorexia, reduced digestion of nutrients, decreased absorption of digested nutrients and changes in metabolism results in lower body weight gain. In an experimental infection model, Adams et al. (1996a) quantified the effect of an *E. acervulina* infection on body-weight gain, feed intake an feed conversion in broiler chickens (table 1).

In experiment 1, two infection doses were used. Shortly after infection with both doses *E. acervulina*, body-weight gain and feed intake were reduced. Feed conversion was increased. The effects were dose related. In experiment 2, one infection dose was compared with a pair-fed not inoculated control and none pair-fed not inoculated control, in order to measure the effect of the infection on body weight gain other than by reduced feed intake. Feed intake is significantly depressed on day 4 and 5 post infections but recovered and significantly increased from day 7 to day 11 (Figure 2). As shown in table 1, body-weight gain in the *E. acervulina*-infected group was much more affected than the pair-fed control group, although feed intake was the same. The consequence of this is that beside feed intake, digestive and metabolic aspects contributes also to decreased body-weight gain in coccidiosis. This was demonstrated by a reduction of the fat and protein digestion and N retention in the period from day 2 to day 11 post infection. Figure 1 illustrates that an infection with *E. acervulina* affects nutrient utilisation in chickens. As the different *Eimeria* species parasitise different

Table 1. Relative effect of *Eimeria acervulina* infection on body-weight gain, feed intake and feed conversion in broiler chickens (from Adams et al., 1996a).

Infection dose*	Body-weight gain (rel.)					Feed intake (rel.)	Feed conversion
Expt. 1	Day 16-23					16-23	16-23
0	100					100	100
280.000	77					86	112
560.000	66					81	122
Lsd	4					5	12
	qua.lin.					lin.	lin.
Expt. 2	Day 18-21	21-24	24-27	27-30	18-30		18-30
0	100	100	100	100	100		100
600.000	103	32	110	111	91		110
0, pair-fed	82	59	125	119	98		103
Lsd	4	25	7	17	5		8

Lsd, Least significant difference; qua, quadratic effect; lin, linear effect.
* Broilers were infected with an oral dose of sporulated *Eimeria acervulina* oocysts on day 18.

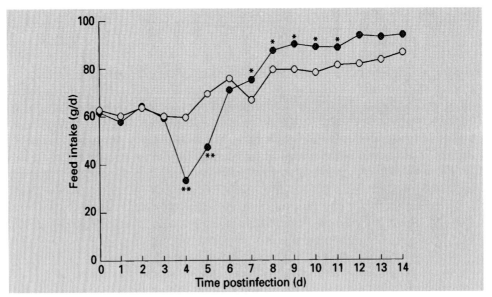

Figure 2. Effect of *Eimeria acervulina* infection on feed intake in broiler chickens.

parts of the gut and are considerable different in pathogenicity, effects on bird health and performance can be more or less severe than with *Eimeria acervulina*.

6.3. Experimental models to investigate coccidiosis and potential

treatments

Experimentally, coccidiosis is a convenient disease to handle, because it is a monofactorial disease, strictly related to the causing agent. Nevertheless, it is important to realise that each species causes a different disease in different parts of the intestine, with different pathological effects, and thus with different effects on feed conversion and health.

Therefore, it is impossible to give a general experimental protocol for all *Eimeria* infections and here only the most important limiting conditions will be described. A more detailed description is supplied elsewhere (COST 89/820, 1995).

Parasites.
Sporulated infectious oocysts can be stored for several months in a 2% sodium dichromate solution at 4 °C. Immediately before infection, oocysts are washed several times and diluted at a defined concentration in water or 0.9% NaCl. The dose of oocysts is dependent of the species and the age and genetic background of the chickens. To ensure that only one and the defined *Eimeria* species is used, oocysts have to be typed regularly, especially after each propagation cycle.

Chickens.
All broiler and layer-type chickens can be infected with *Eimeria*, although there are minor differences in sensitivity. Chickens can be infected at any age, as long as they have not been infected previously with the same species.

Housing and feed.
Depending on the experimental questions, chickens can be housed in wire cages or on the ground, that is previously cleaned with ammonia. The advantage of housing on the ground is that crossinfections can occur, ensuring a repeated infection of all animals. The advantage of housing in wire cages is that faeces samples of individual animals can be obtained. Requirements for the feed are that it is free of anticoccidial drugs, unless it is part of the research. When infected and control groups are involved in the experiment, it is important to separate the groups completely to minimise the risk of unintentional infection of the controls. No specific safety rules apply to *Eimeria*, because it is no human pathogen and is widely spread in the field. Cleaning procedures have to include a disinfection with ammonia.

Infection.
To ensure a homogenous infection of all chickens, they have to be infected by an oral dose of sporulated oocysts. Depending on the genetic background, their age, and the desired degree of infection, the dose varies between 500-2000 *E.tenella* oocysts, 1000-10000 *E.acervulina* oocysts, and 5000-10000 *E.mitis* oocysts. To mimic field conditions, it is also possible to introduce infection using infectious faeces put on the ground or

infectious, oocyst secreting chickens. To obtain immune chickens at least two repeated infections have to be performed.

Oocyst production.
Depending on the *Eimeria* species, chickens will secrete oocysts in the faeces between 90 and 130 hours after infection. At this moment, macroscopic lesions are detectable in the intestine and the lesions can be scored on a scale of 0 to 4 as a measure of the severity of infection. As described above, the different species of *Eimeria* exhibit different degrees of pathogenicity, but within a group of mono-infected animals macroscopic lesions in the intestine more or less reflect the performance of the chickens. Another reliable parameter to measure the infection, is the number of oocysts per gram faeces. Here again, the absolute numbers of oocysts can only be related to the animals performance when the *Eimeria* species is taken into account as well. The main advantage of determining the oocyst number per gram faeces is that it is expressed on a continuous scale, so that small differences can be scored. Detailed information, for example when the mode of action of an anticoccidial drug or an experimental vaccine is investigated, can be obtained after microscopic analysis of infected parts of the intestine using immunocytochemical staining (Jeurissen et al., 2000).

General parameters.
Depending on the severity of infection, chickens will consume less feed and thus show lesser growth than the uninfected controls. The body weight gain of the chickens and the rate of feed conversion form reliable parameters to monitor effects of feed, management or vaccination, and they are easy to collect. Intestinal lesion scores and oocyst output in the faeces supply additional information on the level of infection and the relative contribution of each *Eimeria* species, but these parameters are more elaborate to obtain. Recently, parameters for immunity against certain *Eimeria* species have been developed, such as specific antibodies or *Eimeria*-specific lymphocyte stimulation assays. So far these parameters have not been validated for their prognostic value in the field and they are only used under experimental conditions.

6.4. The use of anticoccidial drugs against *Eimeria* infection

The sanitary practices of in most poultry farms are inadequate for completely eliminating coccidial oocysts, thus protection of all chickens from coccidiosis is not possible. Therefore, the risk of coccidial infection of birds is virtually permanent. Medicating chickens via feed has proved to be convenient, labour-saving and cost-effective and has been a major factor in enabling growers to raise masses of chickens intensively. By far the most extensive use of anticoccidial drugs is in broiler chicken industry, which in 1989 had an estimated world market value of well over US$300 million (Reid, 1990).
Effective drugs to prevent or treat coccidiosis of most types have been available since the 1940s. The drugs are categorised in groups based on their type of compound, such

as ionophorous antibiotics, pyridones, quinolones, guanidines, thiamine analogous, nitrobenzamides, carbanilide, febrifugine, sulphonamides, diclazuril, and toltrazuril. Ideally, a drug should be effective against all *Eimeria* species. However, a drugs efficacy commonly depends on the species, being highly active against some species but inactive against others (McDougald, 1990). The activity of drugs must be seen in terms of specific chemical action, and thus biological action, against developmental stages of the parasite. Ionophorous antibiotics are the most commonly used anticoccidial drug and a short description of its working mechanism will be given.

The polyether ionophores, introduced in the early 1970s, are compounds produced by fermentation of Streptomyces or Actinomadura and the commercial production still depends on large-scale fermentation of these microorganisms. Examples of ionophores are monensin, salinomycin, lasalocid, narasin, and maduramycin. The ionophores act against the extracellular stages, including sporozoites of *Eimeria*. These drugs have in common the ability to form lipophylic complexes with cations, monovalent or divalent or both, and to transport these cations into and through cell membranes. This generally results in an influx of sodium ions that cause severe osmotic damage, evidenced by swelling and vacuolisation of the parasite. A secondary effect is that glycolysis is stimulated in the parasite resulting in a depletion of carbohydrate stores. Ionophores are accumulated by sporozoites before they penetrate host cells, but destruction of the parasite may occur after penetration of the epithelial cells (Chapman, 1993). These ionophores have proved highly effective, but because of their non-specific mode of action, they are also toxic to the host.

Anticoccidial drugs that are added to feed are good preventatives and well-adapted to large-scale use, but the prolonged use of these drugs leads inevitably to the emergence of *Eimeria* strains that are resistant to the drugs. Three important factors contribute to drug resistance in commercial poultry production, First, coccidia are ubiquitous in poultry facilities and they form a large reservoir of genetic variation from which drug resistant strains can develop. Second, the continuous use of anticoccidial chemotherapy provide the basis for changing gene frequency through genetic selection, which in this context may be defined as allowing some parasites to produce more offspring than others based upon their relative sensitivity to the anticoccidial drug used. Third, the coccidial life cycle favours the selection of resistant organisms. Most of their life cycle, coccidia divide asexually and they are then in haploid chromosomal configuration. At the same time, most drugs are active against this haploid stage and therefore efficiently eliminate the more sensitive ones, enabling the more resistant ones to increase in frequency in the population (Jeffers, 1989).

In recent years, poultry producers have tried to slow the development of resistance by alternating different drugs. Two alternation programs are the rotation and shuttle program. The rotation program alternates the use of two or more drugs at various intervals of several months. The shuttle program rotates drugs during the grow out of a flock, with one drug in the starter feed and another in the grower feed (McDougald, 1990).

6.5. Natural defence mechanisms in the intestinal tract

In vertebrates, mucosal surfaces form the largest organ system and as such the mucosal tissues are engaged in a diverse range of vital physiological functions: e.g. respiration, nutrient digestion, and absorption. However, these surfaces, in the conjunctiva, the gastrointestinal, respiratory, and urogenital tracts, also expose large areas to exogenous agents including viruses, bacteria, and parasites. To protect the mucosae, vertebrates have evolved a complex immune system that forms the mucosa-associated lymphoid tissue (MALT). Part of the MALT is the gut-associated lymphoid tissue (GALT). The GALT has two main functions: to protect the animal against enteric infections and simultaneously prevent the absorption of undegraded food antigens and a subsequent harmful immune response.

The structure of gut-associated lymphoid tissues of the chicken.
The gut-associated lymphoid tissue (GALT) of the chicken comprises all cells and tissues along the alimentary tract from pharynx to cloaca. Apart from organised lymphoid tissues, lymphoid aggregates and single cells in the lamina propria and epithelium are also included in the GALT. Organised lymphoid tissue is sometimes located in the roof of the pharynx and further in the Meckel's diverticulum, Peyer's patches, cecal tonsils, and bursa of Fabricius. The Meckel's diverticulum, which is formed around the connection between the yolk sac and the embryonic intestine, is situated at the junction of the duodenum and jejunum (Olah et al., 1984; Jeurissen et al., 1988). Peyer's patches from birds are similar to mammalian Peyer's patches. Peyer's patches occur regularly in the ileum and also at the distal or blind end of the ceca (Befus et al., 1980). Cecal tonsils are located at the proximal ends of the ceca near the ileocolonic junction. The bursa of Fabricius is the central lymphoid organ for B-cell development, and it is generally believed that the main function of the bursa is to provide a site for maturation of the B-cell lineage including the generation of antibody diversity (reviewed by Toivanen et al., 1987; Ratcliffe, 1989). The bursa of Fabricius is located dorsally to the cloaca as a hollow round or oval sac connected to the cloaca by a short duct. This duct provides direct access between the bursal lumen and intestinal lumen, and in older chickens the bursa can function as part of the GALT. At the age of about 4 weeks, the lymphoid system of chicken is fully matured.
During embryonic and postnatal development of chickens, most organised lymphoid tissues begin to develop independently of antigen stimulation, because they can be found at predicted sites before hatching. However, further maturation of the lymphoid tissues is antigen-driven, as can be demonstrated in germfree chickens (Hegde et al. 1982). The development of the GALT starts in the lamina propria of a villus. The villus consists of a core of connective fibres, muscle fibres, nerves, and blood and lymph vessels (together forming the lamina propria), the basement membrane, and a layer of epithelial cells. Around this core, the lymphocytes intermingle with macrophages in the lamina propria, and the more lymphocytes that arise in the villus, the more they form distinct areas of T cells and B cells. Generally, T cell areas are located more at the villus core than the B-cell areas (Jeurissen et al., 1994). The next step in the development of the GALT is the formation of germinal centres, which appear in the

T-cell areas of the deep and mid-portion of the lamina propria (Hoshi et al., 1973). Germinal centres contain B lymphocytes and intermingled follicular dendritic cells. These follicular dendritic cells trap immune complexes and preserve them long after the initiation of an immune response (Kroese et al., 1982). The most important function of this antigen preservation is the generation of memory B cells (Klaus et al., 1980).

The lamina propria is bordered by a thick and continuous basement membrane, and situated on this membrane is a layer of columnar epithelial cells. Goblet cells are interspersed between the columnar epithelial cells and are specialised for secreting mucus. Mucus lubricates the lining of the intestine, but also has a protective function in trapping and excluding parasites (Miller, 1987). The columnar epithelial cells can express a variety of cell determinants, e.g. region-specific carbohydrates or lectins (Alroy et al., 1989) and antigens similar to major histocompatibility complex (MHC) class IV (B-G; Miller et al., 1990). Moreover, the gut epithelium is one of the few epithelia that express secretory component, which is necessary for the transport of IgA from the lamina propria to the lumen (Parry et al., 1978). Only a few studies have been done on the actual uptake of antigen in the chicken (Bockman et al., 1973; Befus et al., 1980; Jeurissen et al., 1988, 1991, 1999). In contrast to mammalian GALT, the epithelium covering the avian GALT is not always containing specialised epithelial cells, the so-called M-cells. Nevertheless, the epithelial cells of the GALT in the chicken also exhibit strong pinocytotic activity (Bockman et al., 1973; Befus et al., 1980; Burns et al., 1986; Jeurissen et al., 1999).

The mucosal immune response.
The ability of the gut mucosal immune system to respond effectively and flexibly to ever-changing food antigens and ingested micro-organisms is remarkable. However, at the same time this system also appears to be limited in the magnitude of its response to any single antigen. This limitation is in contrast to the systemic immune system, which can respond vigorously to relatively rare encounters with non-self antigens. Many factors influence the expression of mucosal immunity to a specific antigen, but a very important one in disease models is the antigen itself, whether it is a live replicating antigen or a dead antigen. Other factors are the route, frequency, dose, and timing of antigen administration; whether administration is mucosal or parenteral; previous experience to the same or cross-reacting antigen at the mucosal site; the species; the genetic background of the host; current infections; the nutritional status and the diet of the host; and hormones and stress.

Vaccines against enteric infections will be successful when they are able to stimulate the local gut mucosal immune system and generate either specific cytotoxic T lymphocytes or a specific secretory immunoglobulin A (sIgA) immune response. Because the mechanism of protection is different for each disease (cytotoxic T lymphocytes, IgA, or a combination of both), it is not possible to give a general indication of the optimal functioning of the intestine. Mucosal vaccines are usually administered by the oral route rather than parenterally (Holmgren et al., 1992). Effective mucosal immunogens appear to have certain characteristics: they are not degraded in the digestive tract, they may have adjuvant immunomodulating activity, and they bind to or penetrate the intestinal epithelium. Although the epithelium restricts the penetration of antigen from the intestinal lumen, it is an incomplete barrier to macromolecules and particulate material. Several ways of antigen uptake have been described in mammals (Nicklin, 1987). Non-specific uptake of antigen can occur at the tips of villi, where epithelial cells are extruded, or via broken tight junctions between epithelial cells. Furthermore, all epithelial cells are capable of non-specific uptake of antigens via pinocytosis, after which antigens are degraded in phagolysosomes.

In addition, specific uptake of antigens can occur by binding to specific receptors that mediate uptake. This has been demonstrated for the uptake of bacterial toxins like cholera toxin (Yamamoto et al., 1988), and for viruses like HIV-1 (Yahi et al., 1992). This form of uptake can bypass lysosomal digestion and is therefore more effective in transporting antigens to the underlying tissues (Nicklin, 1987). Moreover, specialised epithelial cells exist to facilitate access of antigens from the lumen into intestinal lymphoid tissue. These clusters of specialised epithelial cells have been found overlying GALT. At these sites the epithelium contains many intestinal epithelial cells with a well-developed microvillous border and follicle-associated epithelial (FAE) or microfold (M) cells. Morphological features of M cells, like short blunt microvilli and the absence of lysosomal organelles, support the view that these cells transport antigen from the lumen to the underlying lymphoid tissue (Walker, 1981).

6.6. Specific immunity developed during *Eimeria* infection

After oral uptake of *Eimeria* oocyst, the chicken will defend itself against infection in several ways. First, the natural resistance in the form of pH, enzymes, inflammatory factors, etc, will limit the number of viable sporozoites that reach the site of infection. When infection is established, the specific defence will be developed in the form of specific antibodies and specific cellular immunity. Studies on the kinetics of the humoral response have shown that antibodies first appear a week after infection, reach a peak at about 4 weeks and then decline (Davis, 1981). The effects of specific antibodies on the production of oocysts after challenge is however limited. Furthermore, studies in bursectomised chickens have demonstrated that these chickens can be fully protected against *Eimeria*, although they do not produce any specific antibodies (Lillehoj, 1987). Therefore, much research has been dedicated to the cellular actions and interactions that occur locally in the intestine after *Eimeria* infection. In our research group, we have used immunocytochemical staining of cryostat sections of the intestine to examine the contribution of certain cell populations at various time points after primary or secondary infection. In short, the results were as follows.

Once sporozoites arrive in the lamina propria, their distribution within the villus differs markedly in naive and immune chickens. In naive chickens sporozoites were able to reach the crypt epithelium, where they developed into subsequent stages (Figure 3). However, in immune chickens significantly fewer sporozoites reached the crypts, and schizont formation was inhibited. Since we also found that sporozoites

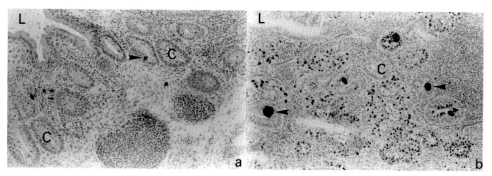

Figure 3. Infection of the cecum of a naive chicken by E.tenella. a: At 8-24 hours after infection, sporozoites migrate from the tips of the villi (small arrows) through the lamina propria to the crypts (large arrow) for further development. b: At 48-72 hours after infection, large schizonts (arrows) and small merozoites have infected large areas of the epithelium.

had penetrated the villus epithelium in equal numbers in naive and immune chickens, we concluded that in immune chickens sporozoites are inhibited by lamina propria leucocytes (Jeurissen et al., 1989; Vervelde et al., 1995a).

In further studies using immunocytochemical staining and semi-quantitative examination, the effects of *Eimeria* infection on the presence and phenotype of lamina propria leucocytes was compared in naive and immune chickens (Vervelde et al., 1996). During the first days of a primary infection, macrophages, granulocytes, and lymphocytes infiltrated massively the lamina propria. Sporozoites that had not reached the crypt epithelium 48 h after intracecal inoculation were often detected within or surrounded by macrophages (Figure 4), suggesting that these cells can moderate the intensity of a primary infection. During this period, the number of CD4+ T cells increased dramatically and outnumbered the CD8+ T cells. Although large numbers of these cells were detected, they were not in close contact with sporozoites (Figure 3). CD4+ T cells were later detected in heavily infected areas where numerous schizonts were developing, indicating that these cells play a role in the induction of the immunity. In conclusion, the primary infection with *Eimeria* activates an (immunological) cascade of defence mechanisms. Different leucocyte subpopulations are attracted to the inflammation site, of which activated macrophages may modulate the severity of infection, whereas CD4+ T cells may act as inducers of an effective immune response.

In contrast to the immune system of naive chickens, which is not able to inhibit the life-cycle of *E.tenella*, the immune system of repeatedly infected immune chickens can almost completely block proliferation of the parasites. In our studies, most sporozoites were inhibited in the lower half of the lamina propria within 48 h after intracecal challenge. These sporozoites could apparently not reach the crypt epithelium anymore. During that time, leucocytes had rapidly infiltrated the lamina propria of immune chickens. Moreover, in contrast to naive chickens, there were more CD8+ than CD4+ T cells. To identify which cells are directly involved in inhibiting sporozoites in the

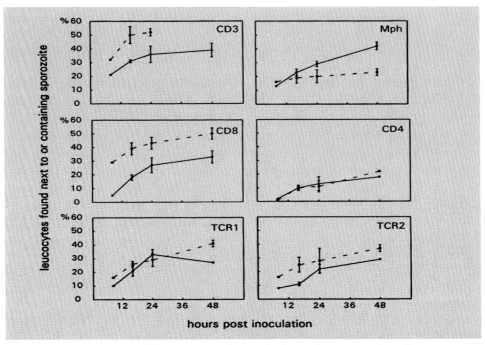

Figure 4. Percentage of leucocyte subpopulations that were found next to or containing an *E.tenella* sporozoite. Values represent the mean ± SEM. Statistically significant differences between naive (solid line) and immune (dotted line) chickens were found after staining of CD3-positive T cells (p<0.001), CD8-positive T cells (p<0.0001), T-cell receptor 2 (TCR2)-positive cells (p<0.015, and macrophages (Mph; p<0.015).

lamina propria, we investigated the phenotype of leucocytes that contained a sporozoite or were located next to a sporozoite (Figure 3). While in naive chickens, many sporozoites were detected within or next to macrophages in the lamina propria, in immune chickens significantly more sporozoites were detected within or next to T cells, especially CD8$^+$ T cells. Our results suggest that more than one cell population is involved in inhibiting the development of sporozoites in the lamina propria of immune chickens, thus that more than one effector mechanism is involved in protective immunity. More research is needed to examine whether CD8$^+$ T cells inhibit sporozoites directly or indirectly by releasing cytokines that activate other cells or alter sporozoite-infected cells into killer cells. The last hypothesis that the effects are indirectly mediated via cytokines, has been strengthened by more recent results that chicken peripheral blood leucocytes of *E.tenella* infected chickens produce interferon-γ after in vitro restimulation (Breed et al., 1997). In addition, interferon-γ has been shown to inhibit in vitro development of E.tenella in chicken fibroblasts and macrophages (Dimier et al., 1998). Treatment of chickens with recombinant interferon-γ preceeding infection with *E.acervulina* has been shown to decrease the negative effect of infection on weight gain (Lowenthal et al., 1997).

6.7. Vaccination against *Eimeria* infection

Several factors suggest that coccidiosis in poultry is a disease very suitable to control by vaccines. First, *Eimeria* infections induce a protective immunity that develops quickly and is extremely strong for some species. Second, the infections are strongly host specific. Third, antigenic variation of the type seen in malarial parasites and trypanosomes has not been described for *Eimeria*. In spite of these positive factors, there are only three short moments during the development of *Eimeria* parasites when the chicken immune system can inhibit the development. The first is when the sporozoite searches for a site of penetration and then actually binds to the epithelium. The second is when the sporozoite is in the villus epithelium inside and amongst intra-epithelial leucocytes. The third is during its passage through the lamina propria to the crypt epithelium. From then on, the parasites do not come into physical contact with cells of the chicken immune system anymore, so there is little possibility for immunological intervention. Attempts to stimulate protective immunity with non-viable material have not been successful. In the world-wide research on coccidial vaccines therefore two main streams can be recognised: vaccines based on the use of wildtype or attenuated *Eimeria* strains, and vaccines based on recombinant viral or bacterial vectors.

Vaccines consisting of viable *Eimeria* oocysts are used mainly during the rearing of breeding stock of both broilers and layer-type chickens. The practical use of this type of coccidiosis vaccines has been reviewed recently by Chapman (2000). These vaccines are generally applied when the chickens are about one week of age, although there is a trend towards earlier vaccination, and they are administered via drinking water or feed. The vaccines Coccivac D/B and Immucox contain a mixture of non-attenuated wild-type strains of *Eimeria*. The numbers of oocysts are calculated so that if they are administered in the correct dose, pathogenic effects should not be observed. The vaccines Livacox T/D and Paracox contain mixtures of attenuated strains that have been selected for reduced or absence of pathogenicity. Two approaches have been used to attenuate virulent strains: serial passage in embryonated eggs, and repeated selection for early development of oocysts in the chicken (precocious lines). Compared with the parental lines, precocious lines have a deletion in terminal generations of schizonts with subsequent reduction in reproductive capabilities and thus in epithelial damage. Because immunological protection against *Eimeria* is highly species specific, a selection of species has been incorporated in these vaccines that varies from only two species (*E.tenella* and *E.acervulina* in Livacox D) up to 8 species in Coccivac D (*E.acervulina*, *E.brunetti*, *E.maxima*, *E.mitis*, *E.mivati*, *E.necatrix*, *E.praecox*, and *E.tenella*). The decision how many species should be included in the vaccine chosen for a certain flock, should be dependent on a careful assessment of the risk of exposure to each of the species. The use of a vaccine comprising *Eimeria* species new for that flock, will lead to the introduction of new species in the local environment. The major risk of vaccines based on wild-type strains is the remaining pathogenicity and thus disease as the progeny of the vaccine strains recycle through the flock and encountering non-immune chickens. This risk is practically non-existent with the attenuated vaccines, but they have their own drawbacks. Although precocious lines have retained most of their immunogenicity, antigenic diversity within a species may cause potential problems in the field and some vaccines therefore comprise two attenuated strains of an *Eimeria* species (Shirley, 1993). Furthermore, the genetic stability of attenuation must be unequivocal. Cross-fertilisation was demonstrated between precocious and wild-type *E.tenella* and *E.acervulina* and although the trait of precocious development was stable, this item remains a point of worry (Jeffers, 1976; Sutton et al., 1986).

Although the live oocyst-based vaccines are successful in the field, it is not certain yet that they will fulfil market requirements for control of coccidiosis in intensive broiler production because of the high costs of production. Therefore, much effort is being generated to develop genetically engineered vaccines. In the last decade, many reports have been published in which partial or complete protection against challenge infection is claimed after immunisation with recombinant antigens (Jenkins et al., 1991; Vermeulen et al., 1993). Furthermore passive immunisation with anti-idiotypic antibodies (Bhogal et al., 1988), monoclonal antibodies (Wallach et al., 1990), hyperimmune bovine colostrum (Fayer et al., 1992), and maternal immunisations as a means of providing protection have been described (Wallach et al., 1990). In view of the fact that protection against coccidiosis is more related to T-cell immunity than to antibody-based immunity, genetically engineered vaccines seem more promising. The essential topics in the development of this type of vaccines are the choice of the candidate antigens derived from a certain developmental stage of the parasite and the choice of the vector. At this moment, no genetically engineered vaccines against coccidiosis are available for use in the field and therefore they will not be discussed in detail.

6.8. Dietary modulation of susceptibility to coccidiosis

Dietary interaction with coccidiosis is not a new area of interest. Many reports on dietary influence on the course of the infection are found in the early literature. Already in 1917, Beach reported success in controlling coccidiosis of chickens by dietary regulation consisting of feeding liberally with buttermilk and sparingly with mash, combined with strict sanitation. But along with the development of efficient low-cost anticoccidial drugs, interest in dietary modulations waned. However, with the increasing development of resistance of the *Eimeria* species to all anticoccidial drugs used, this area has recently attracted renewed interest.

Chicken live weight and feed utilization are generally considered to be the most sensitive and relevant parameters when studying the impact of coccidial infections under controlled experimental conditions. Intestinal lesion scores and oocyst output are valuable to record infection levels and to determine the relative impact of each *Eimeria* species. The information about the effects of coccidiosis is essential for the formulation of diets that are capable of improving the performance of *Eimeria* challenged birds. First, by modulating the resistance to the disease and second, by modulating the resilience to the disease. Resistance refers to the capacity of a variety of anatomical and physiological systems, including the immune system, to exclude pathogens. Resilience refers to the capacity of the bird to maintain productivity during an infectious challenge (Ter Huurne et al., 1999). Dietary modulation of resistance and resilience are not always independent as nutrients may affect both aspects.

6.8.1. Dietary modulation of resistance

The concept of healthy foods in human nutrition in order to prevent diseases has blown over to animal nutrition, especially after the start of the discussion about the development of resistance against dietary antibiotics. A summery of results described in literature to modulate poultry diets to increase resistance against coccidiosis will be given.

Vitamins and trace elements
Resistance or defence to *Eimeria* infection is determined by specific and non-specific responses. The specific response is determined by the bird's immune status and can be enhanced by vaccination. Nutrition may also influence the immune status and thus the resistance to *Eimeria* infections. Several vitamins have been reported to be involved. Vitamin A exerts a specific action on the formation, maintenance and regeneration of epithelial tissue, and Erasmus et al. (1960) showed that vitamin A deficiency was a predisposing factor for coccidiosis in chickens. Vitamin E generally enhances the viability and immune response of poultry, and has been shown to improve resistance to coccidiosis (El-Boushy, 1988; Colnago et al., 1984a). Vitamin C is known to possess immunity enhancing effects in chickens and positive effects on bird performance during coccidial challenge have been observed (Attia et al, 1979). Of the trace minerals, selenium also play a major role in the development and maintenance of the immune system, and Colnago et al (1984a,b) showed that immunity of chickens against coccidiosis was enhanced by a dietary level of selenium higher than nutritionally adequate. Waldenstedt et al. (2000) found that feeding a diet with an extra supplement of vitamins A, C, D3, K3 and selenium at levels higher than normally used in commercially diets had no beneficial effect on the performance of chickens with a mixed subclinical *E.tenella* and *E.maxima* infection. Performance in these birds was actually poorer than in birds fed the control diet, though not significantly. In the same study, birds given a diet supplemented with the putative B-vitamin p-aminobenzoic acid had the highest live weights, even though not statistically significant. p-Aminobenzoic acid, in the past classified as a B-vitamin but being a part of folic acid, has been shown to influence development of *E.tenella* and *E.acervulina* infections (Warren, 1968). Waldenstedt concluded that this result may warrant further studies on the effects of giving dietary p-aminobenzoic acid supplement to chickens during coccidial infections.
In summary, vitamins and trace minerals are not of practical relevance in the susceptibility to *Eimeria* infections as effects are mainly seen in comparison with vitamin deficient diets.

Omega-3 fatty acids
As early as 1938, Murphy et al. showed that fish liver oil exerted a favourable control action on the course of coccidiosis. Recently, Allen et al., (1996) found that oxidative stress may decrease pathogenicity of some species of *Eimeria* parasites. So the link with fish oil was made as it has a high omega-3 fatty acid content and are very sensitive to oxidation. Allen et al. (1996), Danforth et al. (1997) and Korver et al. (1997) verified that diets rich in omega-3 fatty acids reduce the pathological effects (gut lesion score) of *E.tenella* infections. The suggested mode of action is that the omega-3 fatty acids infiltrate tissues of the parasite which become more susceptible to oxidative attack by phagocytic cells. Additionally, omega-3 fatty acids have shown to enhance immune response. However, effects on bird performance showed little if any response, while this parameter is of most importance in poultry production.

Betaine
A compound with presumed effects on resistance as well as resilience to coccidiosis is betaine. Betaine is a tertiary amine formed by oxidation of choline. For this reason it can replace choline, which can be (depending on the formulation) very corrosive to vitamins in premixes for broiler diets. Betaine is present in most living organisms and is concentrated in high levels in the sugar beet, from which it can be extracted. Studies have shown that, when added to the diet, betaine, in combination with the ionophore anticoccidial drug salinomycin, has a positive effect on bird performance during coccidiosis (Virtanen et al., 1993; Augustine et al., 1997).
Waldenstedt et al. (1999) found that betaine as a single feed supplement significantly improved chicken live weight, and tended to reduce FCR during a coccidial challenge. When used in combination with the ionophore anticoccidial drug narasin, betaine showed no effects on bird performance when *E.tenella* was the major pathogenic species. The mode of action is not completely comprehended, but Augustine et al. (1997) suggest that betaine may contribute to the improved performance of coccidia-infected chickens directly, by partial inhibition of coccidial invasion and development, and indirectly, by support of intestinal structure and function in the presence of coccidial infection. The discrepancy between the results of Waldenstedt (1999) and Augustine et al. (1997) may be explained by the differences in magnitude of effects of betaine on invasion and development of the different *Eimeria* species. Overall, Waldenstedt (1999) concluded that the possible potential of betaine on chicken performance during coccidiosis needs to be verified in controlled field trials.

Whole wheat and particle size
Feeding of whole wheat to chickens as a supplement to a standard pelleted feed is quite common in Europe as a means of decreasing feed costs. This practice fits close to the nature of chicks as seed eaters, and it is therefore not surprisingly that healthier birds may be seen in poultry production. Cummings (1992) reported a decreased oocyst output in *Eimeria*-infected chickens fed a high protein concentrate with whole wheat supplement as compared with a conventional broiler diet. This result was suggested to be due to a better developed gizzard, which was presumed to destroy the parasites. Whole wheat increases gizzard activity (Scholtyssek et al., 1983) and would

possibly give a better natural resistance to coccidiosis. On the other hand, it should also be considered that, among other stimuli, the grinding action of the gizzard plays an important role in breaking up the oocysts and thus triggering the release of sporocysts and sporozoites (Fernando, 1990). The results of Waldenstedt et al. (1998) fits more in this hypotheses as in their experiments whole wheat supplementation up to 30 % at 3 weeks of age did not have a significant positive effect on the performance of broiler chickens experimentally infected with either *E.tenella* or *E.maxima*. Also the number of oocysts shed or mean intestinal lesion score did not differ between diets. The conclusion is that feeding whole grains fits well with the nature of chicks but effects on resistance to coccidiosis warrants further research for firm conclusions. In practice, raw materials for broiler diets are grinded and in this way it is possible to influence particle size distribution of the feed instead of adding whole wheat. So the conclusion for whole grains can be translated to compound feed in terms of particle size distribution

Dietary protein source and level
Results by Britton et al. (1964) showed that mortality from coccidiosis was lower among groups of chickens fed a protein-free diet for 48 hours than among chickens fed a normal protein diet. This difference was believed to be attributable to the reduced level of pancreatic juices in the chicken intestine at low protein diets, since chymotrypsin is necessary for excystation of sporozoites from sporocysts (Chapman, 1978). So Waldenstedt (2000) gave chickens a diet with a low crude protein content, but supplemented with the amino acids methionine, lysine and threonine to the same level as in the control diet. However, there seemed to be no positive effect during coccidial infection, as growth rate was depressed in birds given the low crude protein diet, in comparison with the control diet. This also implies that other amino acids, apart from methionine, lysine and threonine added, were limiting chicken growth. From the results of this study it seems that an effect on oocyst excystation would only be excerted during a very low secretion of chymotrypsin. Such a low level of enzyme secretion would most likely negatively affect protein digestion in the intestine, and would therefore not be applicable in commercial broiler production.
Another way to reduce (chymo)trypsin activity in the intestine is to add trypsin inhibitors to the diet for example in the quality of raw soybeans. Accordingly, Mathis et al. (1995) confirmed that coccidiosis in chickens can be reduced with dietary raw soybeans. However, the reduction in body weight gains by trypsin inhibitors eliminate any practical advantages of dietary raw soybeans as a means of controlling coccidiosis.

Dietary viscosity
Non-starch polysaccharides (NSP) occurring in cereals like wheat are responsible for a high viscosity in broiler diets. Addition of enzymes, like xylanases, to broiler diets reduce viscosity in the intestine by partly hydrolysing the NSP. The consequence is a higher nutrient digestibility and so bird performance. Morgan et al. (1995) reported additional positive effects of xylanase supplementation on the performance of Eimeria infected birds. They suggested that intestinal viscosity itself may affect the severity of coccidial infections. However, Waldenstedt et al. (2000) concluded on base

of their experiments with carboxymethyl cellulose that the positive effects of enzyme addition on the outcome of coccidial infections would possibly be more related to other dietary and physiological factors, rather than to viscosity itself.
Despite these indistinctness , the use of viscosity reducing enzymes in cereal broiler diets is a well accepted practice today to enhance bird performance.

6.8.2. Dietary modulation of resilience

As important as dietary modulation to resistance of infections in chickens is the capability of diets to alleviate the impact of infections and to minimise performance and uniformity losses. Resilience, the capacity of birds to maintain productivity during an infectious challenge, can be divided in the infection phase and the recovery phase. In the infection phase of an *Eimeria* infection, intestinal damage occurred which gave a reduction in nutrient digestion and absorption. Chicks have also a higher energy requirement due to fever. As gluconeogenesis take place, a need of glucose may be obvious. Adams et al., (1996b) studied the interaction between nutrition an *Eimeria acervulina* infection in broiler chickens. Effects of diet adjustment on fat digestion were measured. Addition of 0.4 g cholic acid/kg to a diet rich in animal fat resulted in increased fat digestion during infection. So emulsification of fat is a rate-limiting step during infection. Replacing animal fat by coconut oil resulted in improved fat digestion during *E.acervulina* infection (table 2). However, replacement of animal fat by soybean oil did not improve fat digestion.
   A better utilisation of medium-chain triacylglycerols (MCT) which is the main component of coconut oil, is the explanation for these results. MCT fats have certain advantages over long-chain triacylglycerols (LCT) of e.g. animal fats. First, water

Table 2. Effect of coconut oil or soybean oil relative to control animal fat on fat digestion an performance after an *E.acervulina* infection on day 18 in broiler chickens (from Adams et al., 1996b)

	Day	Control animal fat	Infection			Lsd
			Animal fat	Coconut oil	Soybean oil	
Body-weight gain	18-23	100	76	89	80	6
Feed intake	18-23	100	89	93	90	3
Feed conversion*	18-23	100	117	106	116	6
Fat digestion	16	100	102	110	110	7
Fat digestion	23	100	9	56	18	31

Lsd, Least significant difference.
* Feed conversion is corrected for differences in metabolic energy.

solubility of MCT is greater, so bile salts are not required for dispersion in water. In addition, MCT may enter enterocytes without hydrolysis as a result of their smaller molecular size. Furthermore, MCT present a greater surface for lipase enzyme action, so hydrolysis is more rapid. Lastly, the shorter chain length of the fatty acids results in more efficient absorption by the diseased mucosal surface (Babayan, 1987).

In conclusion, intestinal damage in the infection phase of an *Eimeria* infection strengthens the needs for a highly digestible diet. Additionally, in order to counteract gluconeogenesis in the infection phase, easy digestible glucose stores in the diet would be desirable.

Of importance in the recovery phase of an infection is the reconditioning of affected intestinal organs and the restoring of their functions. *Eimeria* infections cause intestinal damage, and a quick recovery is likely to be critical for preventing secondary infections and to minimise performance losses. Importantly, coccidial infections can play a role in the development of necrotic enteritis, as mucosal damage caused by *Eimeria* infections has been shown to predispose for clostridial proliferation (Baba et al., 1988). Coccidiosis also increases susceptibility to Salmonella infections (Takimoto et al., 1984). Stimulation of the mucosal regeneration by addition of substances with trophic effects to the feed would be a possibility which needs further investigations (Ter Huurne et al., 2000).

In the recovery phase of an *Eimeria* infection, there is compensatory growth as shown in table 1, attended with a significant higher feed intake (Figure 2). Adjustment of the feed to a higher need of energy and amino acids of the birds is of importance to make compensatory growth possible and so to minimise performance losses.

6.9. References

Adams, C., H.A. Vahl and A. Veldman, 1996a. Interaction between nutrition and *Eimeria acervulina* infection in broiler chickens: development of an experimental infection model. British Journal of Nutrition 75, 867-873.

Adams, C., H.A. Vahl and A. Veldman, 1996b. Interaction between nutrition and *Eimeria acervulina* infection in broiler chickens: diet compositions that improve fat digestion during *Eimeria acervulina* infection. British Journal of Nutrition 75, 875-880.

Allen, P.C., H.D. Danforth and O.A. Levander, 1996. Diets high in n-3 fatty acids reduce caecal lesion scores in chickens infected with *Eimeria tenella*. Poultry Science 75, 179-185.

Alroy, J., V. Goyal, N.W. Luckacs, R.L. Taylor, R.G. Strout, H.D. Ward and M.E.A. Pereira, 1989. Glycoconjugates of the intestinal epithelium of the domestic fowl (*Gallus domesticus*): a lectin histochemistry study. Histochemical Journal 21, 187-193.

Attia, M. El-S., I.M. Fathy and A.M.N. Attia, 1979. The effect of dietary vitamin C on the severity of coccidiosis in Fayomi chicks. Veterinary Medical Journal Cairo Unversity 26, 65-74.

Augustine, P.C., J.L. McNaughton, E. Virtanen and L. Rosi, 1997. Effect of betaine on the growth performance of chicks inoculated with mixed cultures of avian *Eimeria* species and on invasion and development of *Eimeria tenella* and *Eimeria acervulina* in vitro and in vivo. Poultry Science 76, 802-809.

Baba, E., N. Yasuda, T. Fukata and A. Arakawa, 1988. Effect of *E. maxima* infection on the caecal population of lincomycin-resistant *Clostridium perfringens* introduced into chickens. Research in Veterinary Science 45, 219-221.

Babayan, V.K., 1987. Medium-chain triglycerides and structured lipids. Lipids 22, 417-420.

Beach, J.R., 1917. Bacillary white diarrhoea or fatal septicaemia of chicks and coccidial enteritis of chicks. California Station Circular 162, 1-8.

Befus, A.D., N. Johnston, G.A. Lelsie and J. Bienenstock, 1980. Gut-associated lymphoid tissue in the chicken. Journal of Immunology 125, 2626-2632.

Bhogal, B.S., K.H. Nollstadt, Y.D. Karkhanis, D.M. Schmatz and E.B. Jacobson, 1988. Anti-idiotypic antibody with potential use as an *Eimeria tenella* sporozoite antigen surrogate for vaccination of chickens against coccidiosis. Infection and Immunity 56, 1113-1119.

Bockman, D.E. and M.D. Cooper, 1973. Pinoytosis by epithelium associated with lymphoid follicles in the bursa of Fabricius, appendix and Peyer's patches. An electronmicroscopic study. American Journal of Anatomy 136, 455-478.

Breed, D.G., J. Dorrestein, T.P. Schetters, L.V. Waart, E. Rijke and A.N. Vermeulen, 1997. Peripheral blood lymphocytes from *Eimeria tenella* infected chickens produce gamma-interferon after stimulation in vitro. Parasite Immunology 19, 127-135.

Britton, W.M., C.H. Hill and C.W. Barber, 1964. A mechanism of interaction between dietary protein levels and coccidiosis in chicks. Journal of Nutrition 82, 306-310.

Burns, R.B. and M.H. Maxwell, 1986. Ultrastructure of Peyer's patches in the domestic fowl and turkey. Journal of Anatomy 147, 235-243.

Chapman, H.D., 1978. Studies on the excystation of different species of *Eimeria* in vitro. Zeitschrift Parasitenkunde 56, 115-121.

Chapman, H.D., 1993. Resistance to anticoccidial drugs in fowl. Parasitology Today 9, 159-162.

Chapman, H.D., 2000. Practical use of vaccines for the control of coccidiosis in the chicken. World's Poultry Science Journal 56, 7-20.

Colnago, G.L., L.S. Jensen and P.L. Long, 1984a. Effect of selenium and vitamin E on the development of immunity to coccidiosis in chickens. Poultry Science 63, 1136-1143.

Colnago, G.L., L.S. Jensen and P.L. Long, 1984b. Effect of selenium on peripheral blood leucocytes of chickens infected with *Eimeria*. Poultry Science 63, 896-903.

COST 89/820 Biotechnology. Guidelines on techniques in coccidiosis research, 1995. J. Eckert, R. Braun, M.W. Shirley and P. Coudert (editors). ECSC-EC-EAEC, Brussels/Luxembourg, 306 pp.

Cummings, R.B., 1992. The biological control of coccidiosis by choice feeding. Proceedings XIX World Poultry Congress, Amsterdam, The Netherlands, Volume 2, 425-428.

Danforth, H.D., P.C. Allen and O.A. Levander, 1997. The effect of high n-3 fatty acids diets on the ultrastructural development on *Eimeria tenella*. Parasitology Research 83, 440-444.

Davis, P.J., 1981. Immunity to coccidia. In: M.E. Rose, L.N. Payne and B.M. Freeman (editors), Avian Immunology. British Poultry Science Ltd., Edinburgh. pp. 361-385.

Dimier, I.H., P. Quere, M. Naciri and D.T. Bout, 1998. Inhibition of Eimeria tenella development in vitro mediated by chicken macrophages and fibroblasts treated with chicken cell supernatants with IFN-gamma activity. Avian Diseases 42, 239-247.

El-Boushy, A.R., 1988. Vitamin E affects viability and immune response of poultry. Feedstuffs 60, 20-26.

Erasmus, J., M.L. Scott and P.P. Levine, 1960. A relationship between coccidiosis and vitamin A nutrition in chickens. Poultry Science 39, 565-572.

Fayer, R. and M.C. Jenkins, 1992. Colostrum from cows immunized with *Eimeria acervulina* antigens reduces parasite development *in vivo* and *in vitro*. Poultry Science 71, 1637-1645.

Fernando, M.A., 1990. *Eimeria*: infections of the intestine. In: Long, P. (editor), Coccidiosis of man and domestic animals. CRC Press, Boca Raton, Florida, USA, pp. 64-72.

Hegde, S.N., B.A. Rolls, A. Turvey and M.E. Coates, 1982. Influence of gut microflora on the lymphoid tissue in the chicken (*Gallus domesticus*) and Japanese quail (*Coturnix coturnix Japonica*). Comparative Biochemical Physiology 72A, 205-209.

Holmgren, J., C. Czerkinsky, N. Lycke and A.-M Svennerholm, 1992. Mucosal immunity: implications for vaccine development. Immunobiology 184, 157-179.

Hoshi, H., and T. Mori, 1973. Identification of the bursa-dependent and thymus-dependent areas in the tonsilla caecalis of chickens. Tohoku Journal of Expimental Medicine 111, 309-322.

Jeffers, T.K., 1976. Genetic recombination of precociousness and anticoccidial drug resistance in *Eimeria tenella*. Zeitschrift fur Parasitenkunde 50, 251-255.

Jeffers, T.K., 1989. Anticoccidial drug resistance: a review with emphasis on the polyether ionophores. In: P. Yvore (editor), Coccidia and Intestinal Coccidiomorphs, VIth International Coccidiosis Conference. INRA Publ., Paris. pp. 295-308.

Jenkins, M.C., M.D. Castle, and H.D. Danforth, 1991. Protective immunization against the intestinal parasite *Eimeria acervulina* with recombinant coccidial antigen. Poultry Science 70, 539-547.

Jeurissen, S.H.M., E.M. Janse, and G. Koch, 1988. Meckel's diverticle: a gut associated lymphoid organ in chickens. In: S. Fossum and B. Rolstad (editors), Histophysiology of the Immune System. Plenum Publishing Corporation, New York. pp. 599-605.

Jeurissen, S.H.M., E.M. Janse and A.N. Vermeulen, 1989. Lymphoid and non-lymphoid cells in the cecal mucosa of naive and immune chickens related to the development of *Eimeria tenella*. In: P. Yvore (editor), Coccidia and Intestinal Coccidiomorphs, Vith International Coccidiosis Conference. INRA Publication, Paris, pp. 551-556.

Jeurissen, S.H.M., D. Van Roozelaar and E.M. Janse, 1991. Absorption of carbon from the yolk into gut-associated lymphoid tissues of chickens. Developmental and Comparative Immunology 15, 437-442.

Jeurissen, S.H.M., L. Vervelde and E.M. Janse, 1994. Structure and function of lymphoid tissues of the chicken. Poultry Science Reviews 5, 183-207.

Jeurissen, S.H.M., F. Wagenaar and E.M. Janse, 1999. Further characterization of M-cells in gut-associated lymphoid tissues of the chicken. Poultry Science 78, 965-972.

Jeurissen, S.H.M., E. Claassen, A. Boonstra-Blom, L. Vervelde and E.M. Janse, 2000. Immunocytochemical techniques to investigate the pathogenesis of infectious microorganisms and the concurrent immune response of the host. Developmental and Comparative Immunology 24, 141-151.

Joyner, L.P., 1982. Host and site specificity. In: P.L. Long (editor), The biology of the coccidia. University Park Press, Baltimore. pp. 35-62.

Keusch, G.T. and M.J.G. Farthing, 1986. Nutrition and infection. Annual Reviews of Nutrition 6, 131-154.

Klaus, G.G.B., J.H. Humphrey, A. Kunkl and D.W. Dongwort, 1980. The follicular dendritic cell: its role in antigen presentation in the generation of immunological memory. Immunological Reviews 53, 3-25.

Korver, D.R., P. Wakenell and K.C. Klasing, 1997. Dietary fish oil or lofrin, a 5-lipoxygenase inhibitor, decrease the growth-suppressing effects of coccidiosis in broiler chicks. Poultry Science 76, 1355-1363.

Kroese, F.G.M., P. Eikelenboom and N. Van Rooijen, 1982. Electronmicroscopical and enzymehistochemical characterization of immune complex trapping cells in the spleen of different vertebrate species. Developmental and Comparative Immunology 2 (suppl.), 69-74.

Lillehoj, H.S., 1987. Effects of immunosuppression on avian coccidiosis: cyclosporin A but not hormonal bursectomy abrogates host protective immunity. Infection and Immununity 55, 1616-1621.

Lowenthal, J.W., J.J. York, T.E. O'Neill, S. Rhodes, S.J. Prowse, D.G. Strom and M.R. Digby, 1997. Journal of Cytokine Research 17, 551-558.

Mathis, G.F., N.M. Dale and A.L. Fuller, 1995. Effect of dietary raw soybeans on coccidiosis in chickens. Poultry Science 74, 800-804.

McDougald, L.R., 1990. Control of coccidiosis in chickens: chemotherapy. In: P.L. Long (editor), Coccidiosis of man and domestic animals. CRC Press, Boca Raton, Florida. pp. 307-320.

Miller, H.R.P., 1987. Gastrointestinal mucus, a medium for survival and elimination of parasitic nematodes and protozoa. Parasitology S77-S100.

Miller, M.M., R. Goto, S. Young, J. Liu, and J. Hardy, 1990. Antigens similar to major histocompatibility complex B-G are expressed in the intestinal epithelium in the chicken. Immunogenetica 32, 45-50.

Morgan, A. and M.R. Bedford, 1995. Advances in the development and application of feed enzymes. Proceedings Australian Poultry Symposium 7, 109-115.

Mowat, A. McI., 1990. Human intraepithelial lymphocytes. Immunopathology 12, 165-190.

Murphy, R.R., J.E.Hunter and H.C. Knadel, 1938. The effects of rations containing gradient amounts of cod liver oil on the subsequent performance of laying pullets following a natural infection of coccidiosis. Poultry Science 17, 377-380.

Nicklin, S., 1987. Intestinal uptake of antigen: immunological consequences. In: K. Miller and S. Nicklin (editors), Immunology of the gastrointestinal tract. CRC Press, Boca Raton, Florida. Vol. I. p. 87.

Olah, I., B. Glick and R.L. Taylor, 1984. Meckel's diverticulum II. A novel lymphoepithelial organ in the chicken. Anatomical Records 208, 253-263.

Parry, S.H. and P. Porter, 1978. Characterization and localization of secretory component in the chicken. Immunology 34, 471-478.

Ratcliffe, M.J.H., 1989. Development of the avian B lymphocyte lineage. Critical Reviews on Poultry Biology 2, 207-234.

Reid, W.M., 1990. History of avian medicine in the United States. X. Control of coccidiosis. Avian Diseases 34, 509-525.

Scholtyssek, S., M. Seeman and G. Seeman, 1983. Growing capacity and carcass quality in broilers after choice feeding. Archiv fur Geflugelkunde 47, 166-174.

Shirley, M.W. and P.L. Long, 1990. Control of coccidiosis in chickens: immunization with live vaccines. In: P.L. Long (editor), Coccidiosis of man and domestic animals. CRC Press, Boca Raton, Florida. pp. 321-341.

Shirley, M.W., 1993. Live vaccines for the control of coccidiosis. In: J.R. Barta and M.A. Fernando (editors), Proceedings of the VIth. International Coccidiosis Conference. Moffitt Print Craft Ltd., Guelph. pp. 61-72.

Sutton, C.A., M.W. Shirley and V. McDonald, 1986. Genetic recombination of markers for precocious development, aprinocid resistance, and isoenzymes of glucose phosphate isomerase in *Eimeria acervulina*. Journal of Parasitology 72, 965-967.

Takimoto, H., E. Baba, T. Fukata and A. Arakawa, 1984. effects of infection of *Eimeria tenella*, *E. acervulina* and *E. maxima* upon *Salmonella typhimurium* infection in chickens. Poultry Science 63, 478-484.

Ter Huurne, A.A.H.M. and C.H.M. Smits, 1999. Malabsorption syndrome: a model to evaluate intestinal health. In: Proceedings of the 12th European Symposium on Poultry Nutrition, Veldhoven, the Netherlands, 285-299.

Ter Huurne, A.A.H.M., S.H.M. Jeurissen, F. Lewis, J.D. van der Klis, Z. Mroz and A. Rebel, 2000. Parameters and techniques used to determine intestinal health as constituted by integrity, functionality, immunity and microflora. Report ID-Lelystad Instituut voor Dierhouderij en Diergezondheid BV.

Toivanen, P., A. Naukkarinen and O. Vainio, 1987. What is the function of bursa of Fabricius? In: A. Toivanen and P. Toivanen (editors), Avian Immunology: Basic and practice Vol 1. CRC Press, Boca Raton, Florida. pp. 79-99.

Vermeulen, A.N., J.J. Kok, P. Van den Boogaart, R. Dijkema and J.A.J. Claessens, 1993. *Eimeria* refractile body proteins contain two potentially functional characteristics: transhydrogenase and carbohydrate transport. FEMS Microbiological Letters 110, 223-230.

Vervelde, L., A.N. Vermeulen and S.H.M. Jeurissen, 1993. Common epitopes on *Eimeria tenella* sporozoites and cecal epithelium of chickens. Infection and Immunity 61, 4504-4506.

Vervelde, L., A.N. Vermeulen and S.H.M. Jeurissen, 1995a. *Eimeria tenella* sporozoites rarely enter leucocytes in the cecal epithelium of the chicken (*Gallus domesticus*). Experimental Parasitology 81, 29-38.

Vervelde, L, 1995b. Eimeria tenella infections in chickens. To recognize and to be recognized. PhD thesis, Free University of Amsterdam.

Vervelde, L., A.N. Vermeulen and S.H.M. Jeurissen, 1996. In situ characterisation of leucocyte subpopulations after infection with *Eimeria tenella* in chickens. Parasite Immunology 18, 247-256.

Virtanen, E., J. McNaughton, L. Rosi and D. Hall, 1993. Effects of betaine supplementation on intestinal lesions, mortality and performance of coccidia-challenged broiler chicks. Proceedings of the 9th European Symposium on Poultry Nutrition, Jelenia Gora, Poland, 433-436.

Waldenstedt, L., K. Elwinger, P. Hooshmand-Rad, P. Thebo and A. Uggla, 1998. Comparison between effects of standard feed and whole wheat supplemented diet on experimental *Eimeria tenella* and *Eimeria maxima* infections in broiler chcikens. Acta Veterinaria Scandinavica 39, 461-471.

Waldenstedt, L., K. Elwinger, P. Thebo and A. Uggla, 1999. Effect of betaine supplement on broiler performance during an experimental coccidial infection. Poultry Science 78, 182-189.

Waldenstedt, L., K. Elwinger, A. Lunden, P. Thebo and A. Uggla, 2000. Broiler performance in response to a low protein or vitamin supplemented diet during experimental coccidial infection. Archiv fur Geflugelkunde 64, 34-39.

Walker, W.A., 1981. Antigen uptake in the gut: immunologic implications. Immunology Today 2, 30-34.

Wallach, M., G. Pillemer, S. Yarus, A. Halabi, T. Pugatsch and D. Mencher, 1990. Passive immunization of chickens against *Eimeria maxima* infection with a monoclonal antibody developed against a gametocyte antigen. Infection and Immunity 58, 557-562.

Warren, E.W., 1968. Vitamin requirements of the coccidia in the chicken. Parasitology 58, 137-148.

Watt Poultry Statistical Yearbook 1999. Poultry International, Vol 38.

Williams, R.B., A.C. Bushell, J.M. Reperant, T.G. Doy, J.H. Morgan, M.W. Shirley, P. Ivore, M.M. Carr and Y. Fremont, 1996. A survey of *Eimeria* species in commercially reared chickens in France during 1994. Avian Pathol. 25: 113-130.

Yahi, N., S. Baghdiguian, H. Moreau and J. Fantini, 1992. Galactosyl ceramide (or a closely related molecule) is the receptor for human immunodeficiency virus type 1 on human colon epithelial HT29 cells. Journal of Virology 66, 4848-4854.

Yamamoto, T. and T. Yokota, 1988. Electron microscopic study of *Vibrio cholerae* O1 adherence to the mucus coat and villus surface in the human small intestine. Infection and Immunity 56, 2753-2759.

7. Replacement of milk protein by vegetable protein in milk replacer diets for veal calves: digestion in relation to intestinal health

J.M.A.J. Verdonk[1], W.J.J. Gerrits[2], A.C. Beynen[1,3]
[1] *ID TNO Animal Nutrition, P.O. Box 65, 8200 AB Lelystad, The Netherlands.*
[2] *Wageningen Institute of Animal Sciences, Animal Nutrition Group, P.O. Box 338, 6700 AH Wageningen The Netherlands.*
[3] *Department of Nutrition, Faculty of veterinary Medicine, Utrecht University, Utrecht, The Netherlands.*

Summary

During last decades many researchers have investigated the impact of the replacement of milk proteins by vegetable proteins in milk replacers for veal calves. The attention has been focused mainly on soya proteins and to a lesser extent on wheat gluten, evaluating the technical performance, the digestion, the gut motility and morphology as well as local and systemic immune responses.

In many studies, the calves fed diets containing vegetable proteins had lower protein and fat digestion as well as lower mineral absorption. The negative effects of the vegetable proteins can be reduced to a great extent by means of technological treatments .

In this review, factors involved in the relationship between vegetable proteins, intestinal health and the digestion of protein and fat in veal calves are discussed and the effects on the digestion of protein and fat are quantified.

Keywords: vegetable protein, soy, wheat gluten, digestion, intestinal health, veal calf

Introduction

Commercial milk replacers for veal calves were initially made based primarily on skimmed milk powder and animal fat. As a result of decreasing the price support for milkproduction by the EC the availability of skim milk powder for use in animal feed decreased and the price increased substantially. Therefore, there is a growing interest to use vegetable proteins to reduce the inclusion level of skim milk powder. Skimmed milk proteins consist of casein (80%) and whey proteins (20%). Although various types of vegetable proteins are used in animal feeds, the major vegetable proteins for veal calves originate from soya and wheat gluten. Growth performance of calves fed diets containing vegetable proteins generally is lower than that of calves fed on diets containing milk protein as the sole source of protein caused by a negative effect of vegetable proteins on protein and fat digestion and on nitrogen (N) and mineral absorption. Moreover, veal calves fed vegetable proteins are more prone to developing gut immune-mediated hypersensitivity reactions, which can be persistent for months. Other problems observed in practice with calves fed diets containing considerable amounts of vegetable protein are a decreased appetite and dull haircoat.

In this paper we focus on the replacement of skim milk powder by vegetable proteins and its implications on intestinal health and the digestion and absorption of proteins, carbohydrates, fats and minerals. Vegetable protein related effects on post absorptive nutrient metabolism (e.g. amino acid imbalance, reduced N utilization) are not discussed. Parts of this paper are dealing mainly with soya protein as published data on research with soya protein are abundant and published data on wheat gluten and other vegetable proteins are scarce.

7.1. Protein digestion

7.1.1. General

Compared with diets for other species, dietary proteins for veal calves are usually highly digestible. This is, to a large extent, related to the soluble/dispersible nature of the proteins used in veal calf diets. The veal calf industry has a long history of using milk proteins, originating from skimmed milk and whey. The last decades, replacement of milk proteins by vegetable proteins has become an important issue in veal calf nutrition. Although the true protein digestibility of the products used is generally high, there are negative effects related to increased endogenous protein losses and reduced fat digestibility. Research efforts have focused mainly on soy proteins (soy protein concentrate, soy protein isolate, soy flour), soluble wheat gluten and potato proteins.

7.1.2. Quantifying the problem

Differences in protein digestibility between milk and vegetable proteins have to be separated into differences in true protein digestibity and effects on net endogenous losses at the terminal ileum. Information about the true protein digestibility is, however, scarce. Therefore, in this paragraph, differences in apparent protein digestibility (ileal and faecal) will be quantified from literature data and unpublished information obtained from research conducted at TNO Food & Nutrition Research Institute. Subsequenty, this effect will be separated into effects on true protein digestibility and increased endogenous losses, based on available information.

The effects of replacing milk proteins by vegetable proteins on the apparent ileal and faecal digestibility are summarized in Table 1. From this table, it may be deduced that replacing all of the milk proteins in a veal calf diet leads to a decrease of the apparent ileal digestibility of about 8, 10, 10, 20 and 15% for wheat gluten, soy protein isolate,

Table 1. Effects of replacing milk protein by vegetable protein sources on the decrease in apparent ileal and faecal protein digestibility[1].

	Decrease in ileal protein digestibility (abs % unit)	n[2]	Source[3]	Decrease in faecal protein digestibility (abs % unit)	n[2]	Source[3]
From published trials						
Potato protein	15.1	1/6	1	9.4	1/6	1
Wheat gluten protein	8.9	2/18	1,11	3.2	3/47	1,2,11,12
Soy protein concentrate	10.0	3/24	3,4,5	14.8	9/127	3,5,6,13,14
Soy protein isolate	16.5	1/18	7	9.7	2/22	7,8
Soy flour	30.4	2/16	4,9	33.0	8/44	8,9,10
From unpublished trials						
Wheat gluten protein	6.8	3/13	15	1.4	2/15	15
Soy protein concentrate	-	-		11.9	5/98	15
Soy protein isolate	5.2	2/15	15	12.0	1/12	15
Soy flour	19.7	1/ 4	15	27.4	1/ 4	15

[1] Results are extrapolated to 100% replacement of skim milk powder; on average the apparent ileal digestibility of skim milk protein was around 93%

[2] Number of trials/total number of observations on the vegetable protein treatment considered in all trials

[3] Sources: 1 Branco Pardal et al., 1995a; 2 Toullec et al., 1990; 3 Guilloteau et al., 1986; 4 Caugant et al., 1993a; 5 Tukur et al., 1995; 6 Toullec et al., 1994; 7 Khorasani et al., 1989a; 8 Lallès et al., 1995a; 9 Khorasani et al., 1989b; 10 Roy et al., 1977; 11 Toullec et al., 1998; 12 Tolman et al. 1991; 13 Tolman et al. 1993; 14 Tolman et al. 1995; 15 unpublished information from trials performed at TNO Food Nutrition Research Institute, dept ILOB.

soy protein concentrate, soy flour and potato protein, respectively. It should be noted, however, that the results, presented in this table are -to varying degrees- extrapolations of experimental data in which only part of the milk proteins were replaced. In general, apparent faecal protein digestibility is higher compared with the apparent ileal digestibility, due to absorption of NH_3 resulting from protein fermentation in the hindgut. In Table 1, this is, however, not always the case, due to different literature sources used for computing the ileal and faecal digestibility values. When selecting literature sources in which both ileal and faecal digestibility measurements were performed, it appears that the apparent faecal digestibility is 3.7, 2.5, 1.3, 13.7 and 5.7% (absolute) higher for, wheat gluten, soy protein isolate, soy protein concentrate, soy flour and potato protein, respectively, when compared with the apparent ileal digestibility. The difference seems to increase with the N-flow entering the large intestine, and is indicative for the quantity of NH_3 that potentially has to be absorbed from the colon. Obviously, as shown in pigs and veal calves (Gerrits et al., 1999), faecal N output does not only depend on ileal digestibility, but depends also on the quantity of carbohydrates fermented in the large intestine. This may be important for the protein products that contain fermentable carbohydrates, like for example soy protein concentrates.

Based on the ^{15}N-leucine isotope dilution method, the true digestibility of milk proteins has been shown to be close to 100% (Tolman et al., 1996). Consequently, the N-flow at the terminal ileum has to be entirely from endogenous origin (basal endogenous loss). Based on experimental data obtained with milk proteins over a large range in dry matter intakes, the basal net endogenous losses at the terminal ileum were quantified at 2.46 g N per kg dry matter intake per day (Gerrits et al., 1997). Tolman and others (Tolman et al., 1996 and Tolman et al., unpublished data, Verdonk et al. 1998) have been investigating the true protein digestibility of soy protein isolate, soy protein concentrate and soluble wheat proteins (the latter also by Toullec et al., 1998, based on the amino acid composition of the ileal digesta). The results are presented in Table 2. Data on the true digestibility of vegetable proteins are scarce, and the methods used are subject to continuous debate (see e.g. Hodgekinson et al., 2000). Care should be taken when comparing data obtained by different methods.

Table 2. Effects of protein sources on the true protein digestibility and on endogenous N losses at the terminal ileum[1].

	true protein digestibility (%)	n[2]	Source[3]	Endogenous N losses at the terminal ileum (g N. kg DMI^{-1}.d^{-1})[4]	n[2]	Source[3]
Skimmed milk powder	99	3/12	1,2,3	2.46	5/115	4
Wheat gluten protein	97	3/12	1,5	3.28	3/12	1,2,3,5
Soy protein concentrate	94	1/4	3	3.94	1/4	3
Soy protein isolate	97	2/15	1,2,3	3.94	2/15	1,2,3
Heated soy flour	86	1/4	3	4.55	1/4	3

[1]   Results for the vegetable proteins are extrapolated to 100% replacement of skim milk powder; the experiments, however, were performed replacing only a part of the skim milk powder.

[2]   Number of trials/total number of observations in all trials on the vegetable protein treatment.

[3]   Sources: 1 Tolman et al., 1996; 2 Verdonk et al. 1998; 3 unpublished information from trials perfor-med at TNO Food Nutrition Research Institute, dept ILOB; 4 Gerrits et al., 1997; 5 Toullec et al., 1998.

[4]   Values derived from literature sources as indicated, but numbers obtained were adjusted to have the combination of true digestibility and increased endogenous N losses match the apparent ileal protein digestibility of Table 1.

It is important to realize that the figures presented in Tables 1 and 2 largely depend on the specific properties of the (batch of the) product studied and the degree of extrapolation. Process conditions are continuously improving, decreasing the difference between vegetable and milk proteins.

7.1.3. Mechanisms

As shown in Tables 1 and 2, the protein digestibility from vegetable proteins is usually lower compared with that of milk proteins, in part caused by a decrease in the true protein digestibility, and in part by an increase in the net endogenous losses. Several mechanisms are contributing to this effect. As reviewed for soy proteins by Lallès (1993), the decrease in protein digestibility when replacing milk proteins by vegetable proteins is related to (i) an altered passage pattern of digesta through the gastro-intestinal tract, due to the absence of curd formation of vegetable proteins; (ii) antinutritional factors, leading to increased pancreatic secretions into the duodenum; (iii) altered mucosal properties of the small intestine, and (iv) immunological response to protein antigens. These mechanisms will be briefly discussed below. The contribution of each of these mechanisms to the lowered protein digestibility, however, is difficult to quantify.

Altered passage pattern of digesta
The effect of an altered passage pattern of the digesta, which applies to all vegetable proteins, was investigated by Petit et al. (1988; 1989) and Cruywagen et al (1990, 1991). They treated milk proteins with oxalate buffers to loose its curd formation properties and found (not always statistically significant) decreased protein digestibility when curd formation was suppressed. Caugant et al. (1993b) found a decrease (3% absolute) in ileal protein digestibility when comparing whey with casein proteins, which they attibuted to increased gastric emptying of undigested fractions of the diet. In summary, the altered passage pattern of digesta in the absence of curd formation is likely to cause a small decrease in protein digestibility. It is, however, as reviewed by Longenbach et al. (1998), by no means a complete explanation for the generally poorer performance of calves fed vegetable proteins.

Antinutritional factors
Antinutritional factors like lectins and trypsin inhibitors (soy proteins), glyco alkaloids (potato proteins), and antigenic proteins and protease inhibitors (wheat gluten proteins) are involved in lowering the true protein digestibility of vegetable proteins, but also induce increased pancreatic secretions (and thus increased endogenous losses) thus generally lowering the apparent ileal protein digestibility. The extent to which this happens depends on the amount of antinutritional factors. Contradictory results on the impact of different antinutritional factors on digestibility have been presented (Tolman et al., 1993 and Lallès et al. (1996d). The amount of antinutritional factors present in the product, in turn, depends on the technological process used for its production. Furthermore, a decrease in the true protein digestibility per se is likely to increase pancreatic secretions.

Bioactive peptides
Milk proteins contain bioactive peptides like casomorphins, lactoferroxins and phosphopeptides (Schlimme et al. 1996). The effects of the bioactive peptides are related to f.e. the motility of the gastrointestinal tract, hormone secretion (postprandial), mineral and amino acid transport. Orally administered peptides have been shown to prolong gastrointestinal transit time, to exert antidiarrhoeal action and to modulate digestion and absorption processes in the gut (Schlimme et al. 1996). Van Leeuwen et al. (1998) showed that oral supplementation of lactoperoxidase system and lactoferrin during two weeks resulted in lower incidence of diarrhoea, lower colony forming units of *E. coli* in colonic digesta and faeces and longer villi. In vegetable proteins, the bioactive peptides might be absent or present in lower concentration compared to milk proteins.

Altered mucosal properties of the small intestine
Research by Silva et al. (1986), Seegraber et al. (1986), Sissons et al. (1989) and Lallès et al. (1995a; 1996a) indicated changes in gut wall mucosa morphology in calves fed proteins originating from soy flour, and to a lesser extend, from soy protein concentrates and soy protein isolates. Villous atrophy and diarrhoea related to the feeding of heated soyabean flour or crude wheat gluten were also reported by Kilshaw et al. (1982). These effects are largely caused by the factors mentioned under 1.3.2. Montagne et al. (1999) showed that in the proximal jejunum villous length decreased and crypt depth increased significantly after two weeks when calves were switched from a diet based on skimmed milk powder to a diet based on skimmed milk powder and either heated soybean flour or soya protein concentrate. The villous length was restored two weeks after switching back to the skimmed milk powder based diet. Also the specific activity of a number of brush border enzymes including alkaline phosphatase, lactase and amino-peptidase N were reversibly depressed.The negative effects of soya protein can, however, be reduced by optimizing process conditions.

Immunological response to dietary antigens
Studies in piglets and calves indicate that feeding of legume proteins induces immune responses, starting about one week after feeding (Kilshaw et al., 1979; Heppell et al., 1989; Tolman, 1991). These effects are transient in piglets (Miller, 1994) but seem persistent in calves (Sissons, 1989). A large number of studies indicates that humoral and cellular immune responses occur in response to legume feeding resulting into the formation of protein specific IgG, IgA and IgM and increased infiltration of the lamina propria in the small intestine by B and T lymphocytes (Tolman, 1991; Dréau et al., 1994; Dréau et al, 1995; Lallès et al., 1995b, Tolman et al. 1995, Lallès et al., 1996b). Lallès et al. (1996a) concluded that most soy proteins (glycinin, lectin and the Bowman-Birk inhibitor) are involved in the immediate and semi-delayed immune reactions whereas β-conglycinin causes a delayed type hypersensitivity in calves. Based on direct skin tests and in vitro lympho-proliferation tests, Lallès et al. (1996c) concluded that β-conglycinin was by far the most allergenic protein in soy beans. Gluten mediated gut damage (Kilshaw et al. 1982) and immunoreactive proteins in the extract of vital gluten extract (Branco Pardal et al. 1995a) have been reported.

Unlike in man, cellular and humoral immune responses to the ingestion of wheat gluten have not been reported in veal calves. Doherty et al. (1981) (cited by Kilshaw et al. 1982) stated that intake of gluten led to gut damage in human patients with coeliac disease. He also reported that excessive intake of gluten was related to gut damage in healthy relatives of coeliac patients and in immunodeficient patients.

In their reviews Lallès et al. (1998a) and Huisman (1999) suggest that local inflammatory responses caused by cytokines and other mediators in the gastro-intestinal tract could be of major importance, not only for the functionality of the gastrointestinal tract itself, but also for the general health and well being of the entire organism. Cytokines are hormone-like substances involved in cell-to-cell communication. They are released by activated macrophages, leucocytes and some type of enterocytes, and play an important role in maintenance of the selective barrier function of the gut. Increased levels of the pro-inflammatory cytokines can affect feed intake, energy expenditure, protein, fat, glucose and mineral metabolism by modulating levels of circulating insulin, glucagon and corticosterone. Lallès et al. (1998b) concluded that mediators like histamine and platelet activating factor released by mast cells are involved in immune mediated motility disorders and diarrhoea in veal calves fed heated soybean flour.

Verdonk investigated (unpublished data) the inflammatory response related to the intake of diets containing skim milk protein and vegetable proteins (soy protein concentrate or hydrolysed wheat gluten) but levels of cytokines and nitric oxide were not detectable in jugular blood samples. In contrast, levels of cytokines were increased when lipopolysaccharide was infused i.v. simulating bacterial translocation. This indicates that if feeding vegetable proteins causes an inflammatory response this might be only locally and that the mediators released might be detectable only in surrouding tissues and blood vessels.

7.2. Carbohydrate digestion

7.2.1. Lactose

Effects of replacing milk proteins by vegetable proteins on carbohydrate digestion are not well researched. Typically, a veal calf diet contains 35-45% lactose, being the major carbohydrate source. Lactose digestion in a healthy calf is around 90% at the ileal level (see e.g. Hof, 1980), and virtually complete at the faecal level. Lactose escapes clot formation in the abomasum, and portal appearance of glucose starts within 30 minutes after feeding (Verdonk et al., 1999). Effects of replacing milk proteins on lactose digestion are unlikely, but cannot be excluded as Montagne et al. (1999) showed a 45% decrease in specific lactase activity of the jejunal mucosa of calves when soya protein was included in the diet.

7.2.2. Starch

Increasingly, part of the dietary lactose is being replaced by starch. Up to 15% starch in the diet has been shown feasible in veal calf diets with only a minor decrease in starch digestibility (about 0.3% per percent increase in starch inclusion level in the diet; Verdonk et al., unpublished). At higher levels (15-25%), the decrease in starch digestibility is more pronounced (van der Honing et al., 1974 and Verdonk et al., unpublished). Roughly, 60-80% of the ingested starch will disappear before the end of the ileum (Verdonk et al., unpublished). Visual characteristics and pH of faeces are, of course, affected by the quantity of starch fermented in the hindgut. The composition and the activity of the microflora in the gastrointestinal tract (including the rumen) of veal calves and the effect of dietary protein source on the microflora is not clear. Also the relation between the microflora and digestion and intestinal health in veal calves is not clear and needs to be investigated. Effects of replacing milk proteins by vegetable proteins on starch digestion have, as far as we know, not been investigated. It may be speculated, though, that starch digestion will be affected. It has been shown that pancreatic secretions are among the limiting factors in protein digestion in calves fed soy proteins (Guilloteau, 1999). In addition, increased intakes of (milk) proteins stimulates starch digestibility (Gerrits et al., 1999). The latter was hypothesized to be due to a general stimulation of pancreatic secretions (among which α-amylase) by protein intake (in analogy to reported effects in ruminants, see Mills et al., 1999). Therefore, starch digestion seems sensitive to pancreatic secretions, and the latter is clearly affected by protein source. The extent to which, and even the direction in which, replacing milk proteins by vegetable proteins affects starch digestion remains to be investigated.

7.3. Fat digestion

7.3.1. General

The dietary fat content for veal calves is high compared with pigs and poultry. Replacement of skim milk powder by vegetable proteins not only causes a lower apparent ileal protein digestibility but also a lower apparent fat digestibility in veal calves.

7.3.2. Quantifying the problem

Differences in fat digestibility between diets based on milk and vegetable proteins can be evaluated both on ileal or faecal level because fat digestion in the colon is of minor importance. In this paragraph, differences in apparent fat digestibility (ileal and faecal) will be quantified from literature data and unpublished information obtained from research conducted at TNO Food & Nutrition Research Institute.

The effects of replacing milk proteins by vegetable proteins on the apparent ileal and faecal fat digestibility of the diet are summarized in Table 3. From this table, it may be deduced that replacing all of the milk proteins in a veal calf diet leads to a decrease of the apparent fat digestibility of about 7, 7, 10, 15 and 10% for wheat gluten, soy

Table 3. Effects of replacing milk protein by vegetable protein sources on the decrease in apparent ileal and faecal fat digestibility[1].

	decrease in ileal fat digestibility (abs % unit)	n[2]	source[3]	Decrease in faecal fat digestibility (abs % unit)	n[2]	Source[3]
From published trials						
Potato protein	17.0	1/6	1	11.3	1/6	1
Wheat gluten protein	3.8	2/18	1/7	5.3	3/38	1,2,8
Soy protein concentrate	9.6	1/9	3	10.0	2/47	3,4
Soy protein isolate	-	-	-	5.4	1/51	5
Soy flour	-	-	-	11.6	4/34	5,6
From unpublished trials						
Wheat gluten protein	10.1	2/16	9	9.2	2/15	9
Soy protein concentrate	-	-		9.9	17/98	9
Soy protein isolate	6.4	1/9	9	-	-	-
Soy flour	-	-	9	17.0	1/ 8	9

[1] Results are extrapolated to 100% replacement of skim milk powder
[2] Number of trials/total number of observations in all trials
[3] Sources: 1 Branco Pardal et al., 1995a; 2 Toullec et al., 1990; 3 Tukur et al., 1995; 4 Toullec et al., 1994; 5 Lallès et al., 1995a; 6 Roy et al., 1977; 7 Toullec et al., 1998; 8 Tolman et al. 1991; 9 unpublished information from trials performed at TNO Food Nutrition Research Institute, dept ILOB.

protein isolate, soy protein concentrate, soy flour and potato protein, respectively which is equivalent with a reduction in metabolizable energy content of 5-10%.

It is important to realize that the figures presented in Tables 3 largely depend on the specific properties of the (batch of the) product and the diet composition studied. Furthermore, the length of period during which the diets are fed, the inclusion level of vegetable protein and the age of the calf might affect the digestion and immune response. Process conditions are continuously improving and diet composition is changing, decreasing the difference in fat digestion between diets containing vegetable and milk proteins.

7.3.3. Mechanism

The proposed underlying mechanism in soy feeding involves a lower availability of bile acids for the formation of biliary micelles, which leads to impaired lipid absorption (not only in calves but also in rabbits and rats). Chemically the mechanism is associated with the poorly phosphorylated protein in soy protein compared with the major milk protein, casein, which is highly phosphorylated. The feeding of iso-phosphoric diets containing soya protein instead of casein produces low amounts of phosphopeptides and high amounts of phosphate in the lumen of the small intestine. Low amounts of phosphopeptides will increase the amount of insoluble calcium phosphate which is being formed at the expense of soluble phosphate. The extra calcium phosphate sediment binds extra glycine-conjugated dihydroxy bile acids. A lower availability of bile acids does not only lead to a reduced reabsorption of bile acids but also impairs the formation of biliary micelles, causing a decrease in lipid and cholesterol absorption.

Xu et al. (1998) showed that a diet including soy protein reduced fat digestibility compared to a diet based on milk protein. The soy diet also increased faecal bile acid excretion was three fold and decreased calcium and phosphate absorption. In another study they also found that increased calcium intake depressed fat digestion and apparent absorption of magnesium and phosphorus.

7.4. Mineral absorption

The type of protein in the ration of veal calves may affect mineral absorption. The feeding of soy protein isolate instead of dairy proteins reduced the apparent total intestinal tract absorption of calcium and phosphorus by 6.8 and 8.0 percentage units, respectively. Magnesium absorption was not affected. The negative influence of soy protein on calcium and phosphorus absorption can be explained by the formation of extra insoluble calcium phosphate in the intestinal digesta as mentioned above. When soy protein isolate was fed instead of dairy proteins, plasma and hepatic zinc concentrations in veal calves were lowered. This effect is caused by phytate present in soy protein preparations. Dietary phytate impairs zinc absorption through formation in the digesta of phytate and zinc complexes that are unavailable for absorption.

7.5. The complex relationship between vegetable proteins, intestinal health and the digestion of fat and protein in veal calves

As indicated, the replacement of skim milk powder by vegetable protein can induce changes in the digestion of fat and protein. In an attempt to identify causal relationships in the complex interactions between replacement of milk proteins by vegetable proteins, nutrient digestibility and intestinal health, we distinguish primary, secondary and tertiary factors. The primary factors are intrinsic properties of the vegetable protein considered; secondary factors are caused by the primary factors, but contribute to the decreased nutrient digestibility and poorer intestinal health. Tertiary factors are caused by the primary and/or secundary factors, but also contribute to the decreased nutrient digestibility and poorer intestinal health. For the sake of simplicity, interactions between factors and (negative) feed back mechanisms are not considered. The analysis is presented in Table 4, and the primary, secundary and tertiary factors are explained below.

Table 4. Effect of vegetable protein related factors on fat and protein digestion (– = weak, – – = strong) in veal calves.

Factor[1]	Effect on digestion of		Effect on phenomenon	
	Protein	Fat	Secundary	Tertiary
Primary				
• absence of clotting, emulsifying properties	–	–		
• mineral complex formation		– –		– –
• antinutritional factors	– –		– –	– –
• lower true protein digestibility	–		–	–
Secundary				
• villous atrophy	– –	–		– –
• increased microbial activity	–	–		– –
Tertiary				
• inflammation and immuneresponse	– –			
• mineral absorption ↓ and requirement ↑		–		

[1]   See text.

The primary factors are:
i)   absence of clotting and emulsifying properties increasing the passage rate through the abomasum and increasing the fat particle size (see 1.3.1),
ii)   mineral complexes binding bile salts impairing the formation of micelles (see 3.3),
iii) presence of antigenic proteins and other antinutritional factors causing increased pancreatic secretion, villous atrophy and an immune response (see 1.3.2),
iv)   absence of bio active peptides, resulting in a decreased digestion, absorption and gut development (see 1.3.3.),
v)   lower true protein digestibility (see 1.2).
The secundary factors are the occurrence of
vi)   villous atrophy decreasing the activity of intestinal enzymes, absorptive capacity and increasing the epithelial permeability (see 1.3.5),
vii) increased microbial activity because of increased ileal flow of fermentable carbohydrates present in f.e. soya protein concentrate and increased ileal N flow (undigested vegetable protein and endogenous N).
The tertiary factors are the
viii) inflammatory and immune response (see 1.3.5),
ix)   a changed mineral absorption and requirement (see 4).

Villous atrophy might be very important as this decreases brush border bound enzyme activity and absorptive capacity of the gut and increases endogenous N losses and cell proliferation rate. Moreover, villous atrophy leads to a compromised epithelial barrier function (Branco Pardal et al., 1995b; Mir et al., 1993) increasing the risk for antigen or bacterial translocation and a local or systemic immune response at the expense of amino acids and energy.

In Table 4 we indicate the importance of these factors for protein and fat digestion.

7.6. Concluding remarks

7.6.1. Variability between animals

In addition to effects quantified in Tables 1, 2 and 3, the between animal variability seems to increase when milk proteins are replaced by vegetable proteins. As indicated by preliminary work of Guilloteau et al. (1999), protein digestibility of calves suffering from maldigestion (3 out of 10 calves) was restored by introducing extra pancreatic proteins into the duodenum. In addition, they found that the quantity of pancreatic proteins, needed for normal digestion was higher for soy proteins compared with milk proteins.

Large individual variation in gut permeability, motility parameters, immune response and digestion are reported in soya fed calves but not in skim milk powder fed calves with deviating values for soy sensitive calves. We postulate that increased gut permeability increases the risk of antigen or pathogen translocation causing inflammatory and immune responses. Unfortunately long term assesments to link antigenicity and in vivo gut permeability to macromolecules were unsuccesful.

7.6.2. Length of exposure

Most experiments, especially those focusing on digestibility measurements, are performed over a relative short period of time. Part of the response of a calf to the vegetable protein, in particular the secondary and tertiary responses like immune responses, villous atrophy and increased mineral requirement, may occur or may be increased only after a couple of weeks. Moreover, part of the adverse reactions to vegetable proteins might be related to post absorptive processes (determining the net utilization of nutrients) and might therefore not being detectable on the level of digestion. Therefore, not only short term digestibilty studies but also long term studies investigating effects of vegetable protein on secundary and tertiary phenomena on gut structure and permeability focussing on adverse reactions and post absorptive processes are needed.

7.7. References

Branco Pardal, P., J.P. Lallès, M. Formal, P. Guilloteau and R. Toullec, 1995a. Digestion of wheat gluten and potato protein by the preruminant calf: digestibility, amino acid composition and immunoreactive proteins in ileal digesta. Reproduction Nutrition and Development 35, 639-654.

Branco Pardal, P., J.P. Lallès, F. André, E. Delval and R. Toullec, 1995b. Assesment of gastrointestinal permeability to small marker probes in the preruminant calf. Reproduction Nutrition Development and 35, 189-200.

Caugant, I., R. Toullec, M. Formal, P. Guilloteau and L. Savoie, 1993a. Digestibility and amino acids composition and immunoreactive proteins in ileal digesta. Reproduction Nutrition and Development 33, 335-347.

Caugant, I., R. Toullec, P. Guilloteau and L. Savoie, 1993b. Whey protein digestion in the distal ileum of the preruminant calf. Animal Feed Science and Technology 41, 223-236.

Cruywagen, C.W., G.J. Brisson, G.F. Tremblay and H.H. Meissner, 1990. Effect of curd suppression in a calf milk replacer on physiological parameters in calves. South African Journal of Animal Science 20, 234-238.

Cruywagen, C.W. and J.G. Horn-Quass, 1991. Effect of curd suppression of a calf milk replacer fed at increasing levels on nutrient digestibility and body mass gain. South African Journal of Animal Science 21, 153-156.

Dréau, D., J.P. Lallès, V. Philouze-Romé, R. Toullec and H. Salmon, 1994. Local and systemic immune reponses to soybean protein ingestion in early-weaned pigs. Journal of Animal Science 72, 2090-2098.

Dréau, D., J.P. Lallès, R. Toullec and H. Salmon, 1995. B and T lymphocytes are enhanced in the gut of piglets fed heat-treated soyabean proteins. Veterinary Immunology and Immunopathology 47, 69-79.

Gerrits, W.J.J., J. Dijkstra and J. France, 1997. Description of a model integrating protein and energy metabolism in preruminant calves. Journal of Nutrition 127, 1229-1242.

Gerrits, W.J.J., J. Dijkstra, J.M.A.J. Verdonk, G.M. Beelen and H. Boer, 1999. Effects of ammonia and starch infusion in the colon of preruminant calves. In: G.E. Lobley, A. White and J.C. MacRae (Editors) Book of abstracts of the VIII International Symposium on Protein Metabolism and Nutrition, Aberdeen, UK, 1-4 September 1999, Wageningen Pers, The Netherlands, p 55.

Guilloteau, P., R. Toullec, J.F. Grongnet, P. Patureau-Mirand, J. Prugnaud and D. Sauvant, 1986. Digestion of milk, fish and soya-bean protein in the preruminant calf: flow of digesta, apparent digestibility at the end of the ileum and amino acid composition of ileal digesta. British Journal of Nutrition 55, 571-592.

Guilloteau, P., I. le Huerou-Luron, V. Rome and M. Plodari, 1999. Nutrient absorption is related to quantity of pancreatic enzyme secretion: preliminary results. South African Journal of Animal Science 29, (ISRP) 241-242.

Heppell, L.M.J., J.W. Sissons and S.M. Banks, 1989. Sensitisation of preruminant calves and piglets to antigenic protein in early weaning diets: control of the systemic antibody response. Research in Veterinary Science 47, 257 - 262.

Hodgekinson, S.M. and P.J. Moughan, 2000. Amino acids - the collection of ileal digestia and characterisation of the endogenous component. In: P.J. Moughan, M.W.A. Verstegen and M.I. Visser-Reyneveld (editors) Feed Evaluation - principles and practice). Wageningen Pers, The Netherlands, pp. 105-124.

Hof, G., 1980. An investigation into the extent to which various dietary components, particularly lactose, are related to the incidence of diarrhoea in milk-fed calves. PhD thesis Landbouwhogeschool Wageningen, the Netherlands.

Honing, Y van der, B. Smits, N. Lenis and J. Boeve, 1974. Utilisation of energy and nitrogen from maize and potato starch, pre-gelatinized by physical processing, in milk replacers for veal calves. Journal of Animal Physiology and Nutrition 33, 141-150.

Huisman, J., 1999. Prospects in gastrointestinal physiology in pigs and veal calves. In: A.J.M. Jansman and J. Huisman (editors) Nutrition and gastrointestinal physiology - today and tomorrow -. Papers presented at the symposium held on the occasion of the retirement of J. Huisman, april 1999, Wageningen, The Netherlands.pp 85-103.

Khorasani, G.R., L. Ozimek, W.C. Sauer and J.J. Kennelly, 1989a. Substitution of milk protein with isolated soy protein in calf milk replacers. Journal of Animal Science 67, 1634-1641.

Khorasani, G.R. , L. Ozimek, W.C. Sauer and J.J. Kennelly, 1989b. Substitution of milk protein with isolated soyflour or meat-solubles in calf milk replacers. Canadian Journal of Animal Science 69, 373-382.

Kilshaw, P.J. and J.W. Sissons, 1979. Gastrointestinal allergy to soyabean protein in preruminant calves. Antibody production and digestive disturbances in calves fed heated soyabean flour. Research in Veterinary Science 27, 361-365.

Kilshaw, P.J. and H. Slade, 1982. Villus atrophy and crypt elongation in the small inestine of preruminant calves fed with heated soyabean flour or wheat gluten. Research in Veterinary Science 33, 305-308.

Lallès, J.P., 1993. Nutritional and anti nutritional aspects of soybean and field pea proteins used in veal calf production: a review. Livestock Production Science 34,181-202.

Lallès, J.P., R. Toullec, P. Branco Pardal and J.W. Sissons, 1995a. Hydrolised soy protein isolate sustains high nutritional performance in veal calves. Journal of Dairy Science 78, 194-204.

Lallès, J.P., D. Dréau, A. Huet and R. Toullec, 1995b. Systemic and local gut-specific antibody responses in pre-ruminant calves sensitive to soya. Research in Veterinary Science 59, 56-60.

Lallès, J.P. and R. Toullec, 1996a. Digestion of plant proteins and mechanisms of gut hypersensitivity reactions in the preruminant calf. In: Veal Perspectives to the Year 2000, Proceedings of the International Symposium held 12-13 september 1995 Le Mans, pp. 209-227.

Lallès, J.P., D. Dréau, F. Féménia, A.L. Parodi and R. Toullec, 1996b. Feeding heated soyabean flour increases the density of B and T lymphocytes in the small intestine of calves. Veterinary Immunology and Immunopathology 52, 105-115.

Lallès, J.P. and D. Dréau, 1996c. Identification of soyabean allergens and immune mechanisms of dietary sensitivities in pre-ruminant calves. Research in Veterinary Science 60, 111-116.

Lallès, J.P. and A.J.M. Jansman, 1998a. Recent progress in the understanding of the mode of action and effects of antinutritional factors from legume seeds in non-ruminant farm animals. In: A.J.M. Jansman, G.D. Hill, J. Huisman and A.F.B. van der Poel (Editors) Recent Advances of Research in Antinutritional Factors in Legume Seeds and Rapeseed. EAAP series 93: 219-232.

Lallès, J.P., C. Duvaux-Ponter, W.J. Sissons and R. Toullec, 1998b. Small intestinal motility disorders in preruminant calves chronically fed a diet based on antigenic soya: characterization and possible mediators. Veterinary Research 29, 59-72.

Leeuwen, P. van, J. Huisman, H.M. Kerkhof and K. Kussendrager, 1998. Small intestinal microbiological and morphological observations in young calves fed milk replacers enriched with a combination of lactoperoxidase system and lactoferrin. Journal of Animal Feed Sciences 7, 223-228.

Longenbach, J.I. and A.J. Heinrichs, 1998. A review of the importance and physiological role of curd formation in the abomasum of young calves. Animal Feed Science and Technology 73:85-97.

Miller, B.G., C.T. Whittemore, C.R. Stokes and E. Telemo, 1994. The effect of delayed weaning on the development of oral tolerance to soya-bean protein in pigs. British Journal of Nutrition 71, 615-625.

Mills, J.A.N., J. France and J. Dijkstra, 1999. A review of starch digestion in the lactating dairy cow and proposals for a mechanistic model: 2. postruminal starch digestion and small intestinal glucose absorption. Journal of Animal and Feed Sciences 8, 451-481.

Mir, P.S., J.H. Burton, B.N. Wilkie and E.B. Burnside, 1993. Effects of processing methods for soyabean meal used in milk replacers on intestinal xylose uptake and serum antibody to soybean antigen when fed to calves of various ages.Canadian Journal of Animal Science 73, 191-200.

Montagne, L., R. Toullec, T. Savidge and J.P. Lallès, 1999. Morphology and enzyme activities of the small intestine are modulated by dietary protein sources in the preruminant calf. Reproduction, Nutrition and Development 39, 455-466.

Petit, H.V., M. Ivan and G.J. Brisson, 1988. Digestibility and blood parameters in the preruminant calf fed a clotting and a nonclotting milkreplacer. Journal of Animal Science 66, 986-991.

Petit, H.V., M. Ivan and G.J. Brisson, 1989. Digestibility measured by fecal and ileal collection in preruminant calves fed a clotting and a nonclotting milk replacer. Journal of Dairy Science72, 123-128.

Roy, J.H.B., I.J.F. Stobo, S.M. Shotton, P. Ganderton and C.M. Gillies, 1977. The nutritive value of non-milk proteins for the preruminant calf. The effect of replacement of milk protein by soybean flour or fish-protein concentrate. British Journal of Nutrition 38, 167-187.

Schlimme, E. and H. Meisel, 1996. Bioactive peptides derived from milk proteins: Ingredients for functional foods? Workshop 'Bioactieve eiwitten en peptiden' Oktober 1996, Utrecht, The Netherlands.

Seegraber, F.J. and J.L. Morrill, 1986. Effect of protein source in calf milk replacers on morphology and absorptive ability of small intestine. Journal of Dairy Science 69, 460-469.

Silva, A.G., J.T. Huber, T.H. Herdt, R. Holland, R.M. Degregorio and T.P. Mullaney, 1986. Morphological alterations of small intestinal epithelium of calves caused by feeding soybean protein. Journal of Dairy Science 69, 1387-1393.

Sissons, J.W., 1989. Aetiology of diarrhoea in pigs and pre-ruminant calves. In: W. Haresign, PhD, D.J.A. Cole, PhD. Butterworths (editors). Recent advances in Animal Nutrition. Pp 261-282.

Sissons, J.W., H.E. Pedersen, C. Duvaux, L.M.J. Heppell and A. Tuvey, 1989. Gut dysfunction and diarrhoea in calves fed antigenic soyabean protein. In: J. Huisman, A.F.B. van der Poel and I.E. Liener (Editors). Recent Advances of Research in Antinutritional Factors in Legume Seeds. pp359-362.

Tolman, G.H., 1991. Soya antigens and anti-soya-antibody formation in calves. In: J.H.M Metz and C.M. Groenestein. New Trends in Veal Calf Production. Proceedings of the International Symposium on Veal Calf Production EAAP 52, 241- 246.

Tolman, G.H. and M. Demeersman, 1991. Digestibility and growth performance of soluble wheat protein for veal calves. In: J.H.M Metz and C.M. Groenestein. New Trends in Veal Calf Production. Proceedings of the International Symposium on Veal Calf Production EAAP 52, pp 222- 226.

Tolman, G.H., A.J.M. Jansman, A. Visser and G.M. Beelen, 1993. Nutritional value of soya concentrates in veal calves differing in trypsin inhibitor activity. In: A.F.B. van der Poel, J. Huisman and H.S. Saini (Editors) Recent Advances of Research in Antinutritional Factors in Legume Seeds. EAAP series 70: 205-209.

Tolman, G.H., 1995. Digestibility of enzyme treated soya protein concentrate in preruminant calves. Proceedings of 2nd European Symposium on Feed Enzymes, October 1995, Noordwijkerhout, The Netherlands, pp 85-91.

Tolman, G.H., S. Spanhaak, A.T.J. Bianchi, R. Zwart and E. van Engelen, 1995. Cellular and humoral immune responses in soyabean protein fed preruminant calves. Proceedings Nutrition Society 55, 97A.

Tolman, G.H. and G.M. Beelen, 1996 Endogenous nitrogen and amino acid flow in the terminal ileum of veal calves and the true ileal digestibility of skim milk, soluble wheat and soya isolate proteins, In: Veal, perspectives to the year 2000, proc. of an intern. symp., held 12-13 September 1995, Le Mans, France, pp 191-207.

Toullec, R. and M. Formal, 1998. Digestion of wheat protein in the preruminant calf: ileal digestibility and blood concentrations of nutrients. Animal Feed Science and Technology 73, 115-130.

Toullec, R. and J.F. Grongnet, 1990. Partial replacement of milk proteins by wheat or maize in milk feed: the effect of digestibility in the veal calf. Production Animales 3, 201-206.

Toullec, R., J.P. Lallès, J.P. and P. Bouchez, 1994. Replacement of skim milk with soy bean protein concentrates and whey in milk replacers for veal calves. Animal Feed Science and Technology 50, 101-112.

Tukur, H.M., P. Branco Pardal, M. Formal, R. Toullec, J.P. Lallès and P. Guilloteau, 1995. Digestibility, blood levels of nutrients and skin responses of calves fed soyabean and lupin proteins. Reproduction Nutrition and Development 35, 27-44.

Verdonk, J.M.A.J., G.M. Beelen, A.J.M. Jansman and J. Huisman, 1998. Effect of processing of soya protein on the ileal digestibility and endogenous flow of nitrogen in veal calves. In: A.J.M. Jansman, G.D. Hill, J. Huisman and A.F.B. van der Poel (Editors) Recent Advances of Research in Antinutritional Factors in Legume Seeds and Rapeseed. EAAP series 93: 345-348.

Verdonk, J.M.A.J., W.J.J. Gerrits, G.M. Beelen and A.J.M. Jansman, 1999. Effect of protein source on portal fluxes in preruminant calves. In: G.E. Lobley, A. White and J.C. MacRae (Editors). Book of abstracts of the VIII International Symposium on Protein Metabolism and Nutrition, Aberdeen, UK, 1-4 September 1999, Wageningen Pers, p 47.

Xu, C., 1998. Nutrient availability, with particular reference to fat digestibility, in veal calves fed milk replacers with various compositions. PhD thesis Utrecht University, the Netherlands.

Printed in the United States
by Baker & Taylor Publisher Services